Epilepsy and Intellectual Disabilities

Vee P. Prasher • Mike P. Kerr
Editors

Epilepsy and Intellectual Disabilities

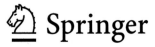 Springer

Editors

Vee. P. Prasher, MBChB, MRCPsych,
  MMedSc, MD, PhD, F.IASSID
Liverpool John Moore University and
  South Birmingham PCT
c/o Greenfields, Monyhull
Kings Norton
Birmingham
UK

Mike P. Kerr, MBChB, MRCPsych, MSc,
  MPhil, F.IASSID
Welsh Centre for Learning Disabilities
Cardiff University
Cardiff
Wales
UK

ISBN: 978-1-84800-258-6   e-ISBN 978-1-84800-259-3
DOI: 10.1007/978-1-84800-259-3

British Library Cataloguing in Publication Data
A catalogue record for this book is available from the British Library

Library of Congress Control Number: 2008929574

Printed on acid-free paper

9 8 7 6 5 4 3 2 1

springer.com

To
Members of our beloved family:
Patrick, Matthew, Thomas, Ajay, Anisha,
and Anjuna

Foreword

Ameliorating the impact of epilepsy and its treatment remains a substantial challenge for individuals with the condition and their families. The challenge however is even greater when the individual has the dual disability of epilepsy and an intellectual disability. It is universally accepted that the occurrence of seizures in a person with intellectual disabilities usually requires a greater degree of understanding of the diagnostic and treatment issues by the treating psychiatrist or neurologist. Recent advances in drug and non-drug treatments, genetics, imaging techniques and a multidisciplinary approach to service delivery have led to dramatic improvements in the quality of the lives of persons with intellectual disabilities who have seizures.

A number of books are available on the association between intellectual disabilities and epilepsy. However, *Epilepsy and Intellectual Disabilities* is the first book to give a primarily intellectual disabilities perspective on this issue. Rather than merely focusing on the seizure disorder per se, this book highlights other complex and interconnected issues of associated cognitive impairment, effects on personality and increased incidence of mental and physical health problems. In my opinion, this book fills a gap in scientific literature.

The editors of *Epilepsy and Intellectual Disabilities* are to be congratulated for bringing together a group of internationally renowned experts in the field to share their knowledge and experience of working with people with epilepsy and intellectual disability. Their effort has culminated in this excellent book, which brings together decades of research aiming to provide an up-to-date perspective on the clinical issues of managing seizures in this vulnerable group of society.

I have no doubt that this book will for many years to come become obligatory reading for professionals managing epilepsy and intellectual disabilities. I commend the editors and wish them all success with their book *Epilepsy and Intellectual Disabilities*.

Gus A. Baker, PhD FBPsS
Professor of Clinical Neuropsychology
University of Liverpool
Liverpool, UK

Preface

This book brings together findings from research and clinical practice with a multi-disciplinary perspective on important aspects of epilepsy in persons with intellectual disabilities. It is important for professionals involved in the care of persons with intellectual disabilities and epilepsy to have a comprehensive understanding of the essential research and clinical issues. Academic books can often lose the vision of a person-centered approach. Clinical practitioners, on the other hand, may not always have the most up-to-date relevant knowledge to provide the appropriate care. This book is intended to fill this gap.

Further, in this book the significant research and clinical aspects of epilepsy in the general population are included and put into a relevant context for persons with intellectual disabilities. Undoubtedly, research and clinical practice are much more advanced for the general population than for persons with intellectual disabilities. It is therefore important that professionals and academics in the field of intellectual disabilities be made fully aware of ongoing developments in the general population, which will more likely than not become important to the intellectually disabled population.

Epilepsy in the intellectually disabled population cannot be discussed as just a disease entity *per se*. The impact on the persons and on their caregivers always needs to be taken into account. Caring for adults with intellectual disabilities who develop epilepsy requires a multidisciplinary approach.

In this book the term *intellectual disabilities* has been used throughout the text. The term has yet to gain universal acceptance, and we are aware that other terms with similar meanings are used throughout the world. For example, the terms *mental retardation, learning disabilities, mental handicap, developmental disability,* or *intellectual handicap* (or variants) are in used in other nations. In this book *intellectual disabilities* is synonymous with these other terms.

Acknowledgment

We are indebted to the many learned clinicians and researchers who have so generously contributed to this book. Without their support and contribution the book *Epilepsy and Intellectual Disabilities* would not exist.

Contents

Contributors

Frank M.C. Besag, FRCP, FRCPsych, FRCPCH
Department of Neuropsychiatry, Bedfordshire and Luton Partnership NHS Trust,
Twinwoods Health Resource Centre, Bedford, UK

Stephen W. Brown, MA, MB, BChir, FRCPsych
Department of Neuropsychiatry, Cornwall Partnership NHS Trust and Peninsula
Medical School, Cornwall, UK

Jennifer D. Dolman, BM, MRCPsych, MSc(Epilepsy),
Learning Disabilities Service, Gloucestershire Partnership NHS Foundation
Trust, Gloucester, UK

Elizabeth Furlong, MBChB, MRCPsych
Department of Psychiatry, Queen Elizabeth Psychiatric Hospital,
Birmingham, UK

Christine L. Hanson, BSC (Hons), RNMH, SpPrCNLD, DipCHS, DipEp
Learning Disabilities Directorate, Bro Morgannwg NHS, Cardiff, Wales

Mike P. Kerr, MBChB, MRCPsych, MSc, MPhil, F.IASSID,
Welsh Centre for Learning Disabilities, Cardiff University, Cardiff, Wales

Ann Johnston, MB, MRCP
Department of Neurology, University Hospital of Wales, Cardiff, Wales

Peter Martin, MD
Séguin Clinic for Persons with Severe Intellectual Disability, Epilepsy Centre
Kork, Kehl-Kork, Germany

Christopher L.L. Morgan, BA, MSc, DFPH
Department of Pyschology, Cardiff University, Cardiff, Wales

Andrew Nicolson, MD, MRCP
Department of Neurology, The Walton Centre for Neurology and Neurosurgery,
Liverpool, UK

Vee P. Prasher, MBChB, MMedSc, MRCPsych, MD, PhD, F.IASSID
Department of Neuropsychiatry, The Greenfields, Monyhull Hospital,
Birmingham, UK

Mark I.A. Scheepers, MBChB, MRCPsych
Learning Disabilities Service, Gloucestershire Partnership NHS Foundation Trust,
Gloucester, UK

Mary Lou Smith, PhD
Department of Psychology, University of Toronto, Mississauga, Canada

Philip E.M. Smith, MD, FRCP
Epilepsy Unit, Department of Neurology, University Hospital of Wales,
Cardiff, Wales

Lathika Weerasena, MBBS, MD, MRCPsych
Department of Psychiatry, Sandwell Mental Health and Social Care Trust, West
Bromwich, UK

Jodie Wilcox, MRCPsych
Department of Psychiatry, Bro Morgannwg NHS Trust, Cardiff, Wales

Sameer M. Zuberi, MB, ChB, FRCP, FRCPCH
Fraser of Allander Neurosciences Unit, Royal Hospital for Sick Children,
Glasgow, Scotland

Section I
Clinical Issues

Chapter 1
Introduction

M.P. Kerr

The frequent coexistence of intellectual disabilities (ID) and epilepsy can pose special challenges to those with the conditions and those delivering care. The considerable crossovers between the two conditions compound these challenges. The first, ID, is essentially a broad term encompassing constructs of intelligence, adaptive functioning, and developmental impact. As such, it can be seen to have biological and social components necessitating an often complex delivery of care spanning education, employment, and health. Epilepsy has similar issues: it is an essentially organic condition influenced by the environment and greatly impacts physical and psychological health. It also contributes to poor social outcomes, and again optimal care requires multiprofessional involvement.

This situation may well be reflected in the strong evidence for the inequality in health care experienced by people with ID. This combination of inequality of health care access and health promotion uptake, along with increased hospitalization and mortality rates, is mirrored, and often exceeded, in those people with ID who also have epilepsy.

The focus of epilepsy management is therefore to address those issues leading to this inequality in health care experience. In this introduction I will use a clinical scenario to show how these issues are linked. This scenario is reflected in the case of John, whom I describe below, and whom you know either as professional, caregiver, friend, or relative and for whom you want to apply or access an individualized care package that includes his wishes and that reduces his epilepsy-related morbidity.

John is a young man of 24 who lives in supported accommodation and whose disabilities include problems with communication, the need for physical care, and frequent seizures. He takes a range of medications for both epilepsy and his behaviorproblems and sees his general practitioner on an "on-demand" basis. He has had limited medical follow-up since finishing his education. In his last review he was described as stable; no plans are in place for further specialist review.

John is not unrepresentative of people with ID and epilepsy. He poses some clinical and care challenges, yet more importantly he may benefit greatly from quality clinical care. There are several key components in his assessment and management, and they are dealt with in this book. I will summarize these after addressing the first challenge John faces: accessing appropriate care.

V.P. Prasher, M.P. Kerr (eds.) *Epilepsy and Intellectual Disabilities*,
DOI: 10.1007/978-1-84800-259-3_1, © Springer Science+Business Media, LLC 2008

✳Access to Care

An individual with this range of issues should be accessing specialist epilepsy care either in neurology, ID psychiatry, or other epilepsy-aware settings. Data from the National Sentinel Audit into epilepsy-related deaths revealed that some individuals transitioning from child to adult services did not in fact transition their epilepsy care, and these individuals suffered epilepsy-related death. To avoid this outcome, John's caregivers or others need to access such services. Such a transition may be further hampered by difficulties that exist in accessing primary care services in the United Kingdom. The caregiver, advocates, or associated professionals may need to make a strong case for referral based on the impact of epilepsy on John's life and the risk it poses to him.

Getting the Diagnosis Right

Specialist services will focus initially on confirming an accurate diagnosis of sepilepsy, seizure type, and syndrome. For John this may lead to a greater understanding of his condition and its prognosis. If in fact the diagnosis is inaccurate he may benefit by reducing or discontinuing medications.

Treatment Issues

John may benefit greatly from a detailed approach to his treatment options; placing him on an appropriate treatment pathway would enable him to understand his condition and the treatment options he may wish to access.

High-quality treatment will involve matching the drugs with his syndrome and seizure types and clear assessment of the potential medication side effects. As discussed in this book, access to surgical procedures may also offer hope in terms of seizure change.

For many people with ID the management of acute seizures can lead to as much improvement in their quality of life as trying to reduce overall seizure numbers because this approach increases social and residential options and reduces the frequency of hospitalization. It is likely that any epilepsy-aware service would address the need for protocols for acute seizure management.

Psychosocial Issues

These issues can often dominate an individual's epilepsy care. Caregiver concerns about behavior problems can lead to inertia in management, as fears of behavior change associated with changes in epilepsy treatment may stop progress on the treatment pathway.

Like many people with epilepsy and ID, John has comorbid behavior problems. This association is dealt with in detail later in the book. A clear and consistent approach to this is likely to offer much to John in terms of his quality of life. Other psychosocial concerns will need addressing. Emphasizing and explaining the impact of epilepsy and its treatment on John's cognitive well-being can help reduce anxiety in caregivers and the family and help establish the importance of treatment. Informing people about the negative impact of seizures while trying to minimize the difficulties in social life imposed by people's fears of seizures can be a difficult challenge. This is most difficult when discussing seizure-related death. However, our position must be to inform patients and families so they can make their life and treatment choices with complete understanding of choices and risks.

Delivering a Package of Care

Delivering continuity of health care will be a major need throughout John's lifespan. This continuity should cover seizure assessment and management yet also be responsive to changes in the care environment. A person with ID who is no longer resident in the family home is likely to undergo many changes in staffing over a lifetime. As for many people, their ability to communicate their health needs will be compromised, and these changes in staff can offer considerable risks in chronic disease management. Such a situation cries out for consistent health care services over an individual's lifetime.Unfortunately this need is at odds with the drive for early discharge. Epilepsy-aware services with a skilled multiprofessional team can at least offer some continuity of care to support individuals like John over the long term.

In conclusion the broad scope of knowledge in this book has at its core the simple presumption that such knowledge improves the lives of individuals. People with ID will benefit from professionals keen to learn and continually expand their skills and competencies.

Chapter 2
Epilepsy: A General Overview

A. Johnston and P. Smith

Introduction

Epilepsy is a common disabling, chronic, and socially isolating condition. Even in the 21st century, an epilepsy diagnosis carries social stigma and affects individuals and their families physically, psychologically, and financially. Despite this, the increasing understanding of its scientific basis, together with advances in neuroimaging, neurosurgery, and neuropharmacology, have given patients with epilepsy and their families greater investigative and therapeutic options and the promise of an improved quality of life.

Epilepsy is a clinical diagnosis; there is no one diagnostic "test." In all people with undiagnosed blackouts, and even in people with an established label of epilepsy, the clinician must invest considerable time and attention to obtain or confirm the diagnosis, to classify the epilepsy, to identify underlying structural causes, and to plan relevant medical or surgical treatment. The ultimate goals of epilepsy management are seizure freedom without adverse medication effects.

Definitions

Seizures are sudden and usually transient stereotyped clinical episodes of disturbed behavior, emotion, or motor or sensory function that may or may not be accompanied by a change in consciousness level. They result from abnormal excessive but synchronized discharges from a set of cerebral neurons. The diagnosis of a seizure is largely clinical and relies heavily on the history and on an accurate witnessed account.

Epilepsy is the tendency to experience recurrent unprovoked seizures. In practice this implies two or more spontaneous seizures in a greater than 24-hour period. A single seizure is not epilepsy.

Status epilepticus is either a prolonged seizure or repeated epileptic seizures lasting for over 30 minutes, without intervening recovered consciousness.

V.P. Prasher, M.P. Kerr (eds.) *Epilepsy and Intellectual Disabilities*,
DOI: 10.1007/978-1-84800-259-3_2, © Springer Science+Business Media, LLC 2008

Classification of Seizures

Seizure classification is still based upon the 1989 consensus report by the Commission on Classification and Terminology of the International League Against Epilepsy.[1] There are two main patterns of seizure discharge:

- Those arising from focal cortical disturbances, causing partial-onset seizures. These often begin with an aura that reflects the functional role of that cortex, e.g., a visual cortex seizure causing a visual aura.
- Those characterized by immediate synchronous spike-wave discharge of both hemispheres, causing generalized seizures. In these, consciousness is lost suddenly and without warning, owing to extensive cortical and subcortical involvement.

Partial Seizures

Partial seizures are either **simple** (retained consciousness) or **complex** (altered consciousness). A *complex partial seizure* may begin with an aura but then progresses to a state of altered awareness with stereotyped behaviors ("automatisms," e.g., lip smacking, fidgeting, plucking at clothing) and sometimes more complex or bizarre behaviors. The seizure is often followed by a period of postictal confusion. The patient may remember the aura but not the seizure itself.

The clinical features reflect the region of seizure origin; the initial seizure symptom (aura) is useful in localizing the event. Most partial-onset seizures arise in the temporal or frontal lobes.

- **Temporal lobe seizures** are the classic complex partial seizures. The aura may be a rising epigastric sensation (suggesting underlying hippocampal sclerosis), déjà vu (typically from dominant hemisphere onset), abnormal tastes or smells, and often unpleasant psychic phenomena. Auditory hallucinations are uncommon and imply a lateral temporal lobe focus. Autonomic features include flushing, pupillary dilatation, apnea, and heart rate changes. Motor phenomena during the seizure include lip smacking, nose wiping (amygdala involvement), hand automatisms (e.g., plucking at clothing; ipsilateral to seizure onset) and upper limb dystonic posturing (contralateral to seizure onset). Forced head turning and secondary generalized tonic-clonic seizures are common in temporal lobe seizures, but imply ictal spread beyond the temporal lobe.
- **Frontal lobe seizures** include a variety of seizure types, reflecting the large size of the frontal lobe. Classic Jacksonian epilepsy arises in the motor cortex and manifests as a "march" of limb jerking spreading from the hand (usually the thumb, reflecting its large cortical representation) to the whole side of the body; postictally there may be a transient focal weakness (Todd's phenomenon). Others may manifest as forced head and eye turning (contralateral to the seizure onset), with arm jerking or elevation (the "fencing position"). There may be

speech arrest or unintelligible muttering (both suggesting dominant hemisphere onset). Seizures arising in the supplementary motor area are characteristically very brief (<30 seconds), frequently arising from sleep, often with retained consciousness, and sometimes with "hypermotor" phenomena (e.g., running, punching, cycling). The surface electroencephalogram (EEG) may even appear unchanged because of the deep midline seizure onset. The combination of bizarre behaviors and unchanged ictal EEG risk the seizures being mislabeled as psychogenic.

- **Occipital lobe seizures** are unusual and present with visual perceptual abnormalities such as balls of light or colors, usually in the contralateral visual field; there may be ipsilateral eye deviation. There is often clinical overlap with migraine symptoms.
- **Parietal lobe seizures** are rare and characterized by lateralized positive sensory disturbance, e.g., tingling or pain.

Generalized Seizures

In a generalized seizure, consciousness is impaired from the onset. The major types of generalized seizures include absence, myoclonic, tonic-clonic, tonic, and atonic seizures

Absences

- **Typical absences** of childhood are characterized by abrupt loss of consciousness, with momentary loss of contact and cessation of activity. There may be eyelid myoclonus, altered axial tone, and even automatisms. The ictal EEG is very striking, showing 3-Hz generalized spike-and-wave (Figure 2.1). The EEG changes, and seizures are characteristically precipitated by hyperventilation.
- **Atypical absences** are more common, more prolonged, have less abrupt onset and offset, and are often associated with myoclonus and changes in muscle tone. The loss of awareness is often incomplete. The ictal EEG shows slow or fast spike-and-wave activity. Atypical absences characteristically occur in children with pre-existing brain damage and intellectual disability, and so may form part of the Lennox-Gastaut syndrome.

Myoclonic Jerks

Myoclonic jerks are brief limb jerks, especially of the arms; they are sudden, usually symmetrical, occasionally violent, and usually associated with a cortical discharge. They occur in several epileptic syndromes.

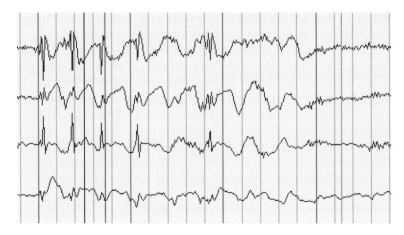

Fig. 2.1 EEG demonstrating spike activity and wave activity

Tonic-Clonic Seizures

Tonic-clonic seizures manifest as loss of consciousness followed by a "tonic phase" (extension and stiffening, sometimes with a cry, cyanosis, and tongue biting) followed by the "clonic phase" (rhythmical jerking of the limbs). There may be injuries and incontinence. Afterwards, patients are drowsy, and report headache and aching muscles.

Tonic Seizures

Tonic seizures manifest as a tonic muscle contraction of the limbs and trunk, with altered consciousness and often a fall with injury.

Atonic Seizures

Atonic seizures are caused by an abrupt loss of muscle tone, and so often cause falls and injuries.

Secondary Generalized Tonic-Clonic Seizures

These seizures are either preceded by a partial seizure or occur without warning (mimicking a primary generalized seizure). Convulsions during sleep are usually secondarily generalized, whereas convulsions on awakening are typically primary generalized.

Classification of Epilepsy

Similar to the classification of seizures, epilepsy classification is also based upon the 1989 consensus report by the Commission on Classification and Terminology of the International League Against Epilepsy.[1] Epilepsies, each of which may manifest as a number of seizure types, are classified according to two characteristics.

1. **The site of seizure onset**. The predominant seizure type is considered (on clinical and EEG grounds) to be either generalized (in a generalized epilepsy) or focal (in a focal or localization-related epilepsy).
2. **The presumed seizure etiology**. This may be symptomatic (implying a known structural cause), cryptogenic (the presumed structural cause cannot be identified), or idiopathic (more than "unknown cause," this implies a presumed genetic cause with seizures of age-specific onset and sometimes age-specific offset, normal cerebral imaging, and expected good response to antiepileptic medication).

Causes of Epilepsy

The commonest adult epilepsies are idiopathic generalized and symptomatic focal.

Idiopathic Generalized Epilepsies

Idiopathic generalized epilepsies take many forms, but the best-known examples are childhood absence epilepsy and juvenile myoclonic epilepsy (JME). The seizure types of JME comprise morning myoclonus, generalized tonic-clonic seizures on awakening, and sometimes absences and photosensitivity, all more likely following sleep deprivation. The seizures typically begin in the teenage years, but the epilepsy tendency persists lifelong. The EEG shows interictal generalized polyspike-and-wave activity (Figure 2.2). The seizures usually respond well to valproate.

Symptomatic Focal Epilepsies

Symptomatic focal epilepsies have many possible causes. The commonest in adults is hippocampal (mesial temporal) sclerosis. The typical history is of an early life cerebral insult, e.g., prolonged focal febrile seizure, followed by a latent interval of sometimes many years before the onset of complex partial seizures, characteristically with an epigastric aura. The seizures are often resistant to antiepileptic medication and the epilepsy may worsen with time, requiring increasing medication doses.

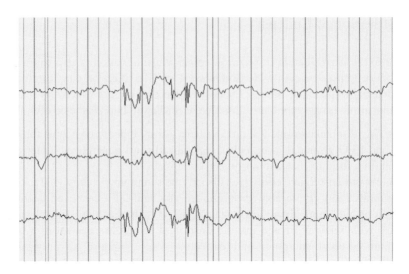

Fig. 2.2 EEG demonstrating polyspike activity and wave activity

Surgery (temporal lobectomy) is potentially curative. Other common symptomatic focal epilepsies include those arising from head injury (typically frontal and temporal lobe involvement), tumors (especially low-grade tumors involving cortex, causing sometimes very resistant and frequent seizures), cortical dysplasias (ranging from minor focal areas with normal intellect to generalized cortical abnormality with severe intellectual disability), and arteriovenous malformations and cavernous hemangiomas (iron products from minor bleeding being potentially very epileptogenic).

Epidemiology

Epilepsy is the commonest serious chronic neurological disorder in adults after stroke.

Incidence

In developed societies, around 50 people per 100,000 develop epilepsy each year[2] (excluding febrile convulsions and single seizures). The incidence is higher in developing countries, perhaps almost double at 100 per 100,000. Contributing factors include social deprivation, malnutrition, pre- and perinatal complications, and an increased risk of conditions with permanent brain damage sequelae, e.g., neurocysticercosis, meningitis, and cerebral malaria.[3]

Prevalence

Five to 10 people per 1,000 have a diagnosis of epilepsy (not including febrile convulsions, single seizures, and inactive cases). The overall lifetime prevalence of seizures (the risk of a nonfebrile epileptic seizure at some point in an average lifetime) is 2–5%.[4] The prevalence is highest in neonates and young children, peaking again in the elderly.

Differential Diagnosis of Epilepsy

The diagnostic possibilities of an episode of altered consciousness are vast. It is therefore essential that all relevant information be obtained before a diagnosis of epilepsy is made, including the identification of potential triggers and provoking factors. The clinical history must include a full past medical history, specifically previous significant head injury, meningitis or encephalitis, a birth history, any history of febrile convulsions, and any family history of epilepsy.

 The diagnosis of epilepsy is clinical and relies on accurate personal and eyewitnessed accounts, concentrating on the circumstances of episode, the preceding aura, the interictal state, and postictal events. A diagnosis of epilepsy is a lifechanging event with potential psychological consequences; the diagnosis should be given and relevant treatment begun only when the there is reasonable certainty. On first contact with the patient all the relevant information may not be at hand; the passage of time can be an important diagnostic tool in avoiding misdiagnosis. The conditions most commonly mistaken for epileptic seizures are syncope (vasovagal and cardiac), nonepileptic attacks, and sleep disorders. Table 2.1 outlines other conditions to be considered in the differential diagnosis of epilepsy.

Table 2.1 Differential diagnosis of epilepsy

Syncope	Vasovagal (see text)
	Orthostatic (autonomic failure)
	Cardiac (arrhythmia or structural)
Psychogenic	Panic attacks
	Dissociative attacks
Vascular	Migraine (especially basilar artery migraine)
	Transient ischemic attacks (especially brainstem)
	Transient global amnesia
Sleep disorders	Parasomnias
	Narcolepsy
Metabolic	Hypoglycemia and insulinoma
	Hypocalcemia
Toxic	Drugs
	Alcohol

Table 2.2 Seizures versus syncope

	Seizure	Syncope
Precipitating factor	Rare	Common
Situation	Anywhere	Bathroom
		Dances
		Pubs
		Queues
Prodrome	Aura	Nausea, sweating
		Visual blurring
		Hearing fades
Onset	Sudden	Gradual
Duration	Minutes	Seconds
Consciousness	Lost	Briefly uncon-scious
		May recall falling
Jerks	Common	Briefly
Incontinence	Common	Rarely
Lateral tongue bite	Common	Rarely
Color	Pale, blue, cyanosis	Very pale, white
Recovery	Slow	Rapid
Confusion	Common	Rarely

Adapted from Smith.[5]

Syncope

Syncope is an abrupt and transient loss of consciousness due to a sudden decrease in cerebral perfusion. It is the condition most commonly confused with epilepsy. Table 2.2 contrasts syncope with epilepsy.

Also, like epilepsy, syncope is a clinical diagnosis, for which an eye-witnessed account is essential. There are two main subtypes.

Neurocardiogenic Syncope

The main form of neurocardiogenic syncope is vasovagal syncope: this is the commonest cause of loss of consciousness. There is usually a clear precipitating factor, such as prolonged standing, a hot environment, fright, or the sight of blood. Vasovagal syncope typically begins with the prodrome of nausea, clamminess, sweating, tunnelling and loss of vision (blurred or black), light headedness, and tinnitus. The patient may look pale and sweaty. In the event itself, there is reduced muscle tone, causing the eyes to elevate and the patient to slump to the ground. There may be a few small-amplitude and brief myoclonic jerks during the anoxic phase, which may easily be misinterpreted as an epileptic seizure. Consciousness is usually regained within a few seconds. Amnesia, drowsiness, and confusion are usually only brief. Injury and incontinence occasionally occur, but lateral tongue biting is very unusual.

Fainting may be more severe if the patient is held upright, e.g., if confined to the small space in a toilet or airplane, causing delayed recovery of cerebral perfusion and a secondary anoxic convulsion.

An accurate history, including the circumstances of the attack and an eye-witnessed account, are usually sufficient to diagnose vasovagal syncope. A 12-lead ECG is the most useful investigation (to exclude other more serious causes of syncope); head-up tilt table testing can assist the diagnosis.

Cardiac Syncope

Whereas neurocardiogenic syncope is fairly benign, cardiac syncope is potentially fatal. Causes include either cardiac arrhythmias (e.g., Wolff-Parkinson-White syndrome, long QT syndromes) or structural heart disease (e.g., hypertrophic cardiomyopathy, aortic stenosis). These require an accurate history, a full neurological and cardiac examination, ECG, echocardiography, and even prolonged ECG monitoring (24-hour or embedded long-term monitoring).

Psychogenic Nonepileptic Attack Disorders

As many as 20% of patients previously diagnosed with epilepsy (often for years) turn out to have nonepileptic attacks.[6,7]

Panic Disorder

Panic symptoms are usually characterized by a period of hyperventilation, dizziness, palpitations, chest pain, sweating, blurred vision, fatigue, parasthesia, and often overwhelming fear and anxiety. Usually they are easily recognizable, though they sometimes may be difficult to distinguish from temporal lobe seizures.

Dissociative Attacks ("Pseudoseizures")

These are psychologically mediated episodes of altered awareness and/or behavior which may mimic any type of epilepsy. Most (non-learning-disabled) adults with dissociative attacks are female (75%),[8] usually presenting in their late teens or early 20s. There is often is a history of multiple unexplained illnesses and multiple investigations, and there may be a history of physical or sexual abuse. Suspicion arises when, despite normal investigations and high doses of antiepileptic medication, attacks remain frequent, sometimes several per day, and even result in hospital admissions and intensive care management for presumed "status."

Features suggesting a nonepileptic event rather than an epileptic seizure include gradual onset, prolonged duration, fluctuating motor activity during the event, and

Table 2.3 Epileptic versus psychogenic nonepileptic attacks

	Nonepileptic Attacks	Epileptic Seizures
Situation	Mostly Witnessed	Rarely Witnessed
Onset	Gradual	Sudden
Duration	Minutes to hours	Minutes
Stereotyped events	Common	Common
Color	Pink	Pale, red or cyanosed
Motor features:		
Gradual onset	Common	Rare
Fluctuating course	Common	Very rare
Thrashing, violent	Common	Rare
Side-to-side head	Common	Rare
Eyes closed	Common	Rare
Pelvic thrusting	Common	Rare
Automatisms	Rare	Common
Rapid breathing	Common	Rare
Consciousness	May be retained	Lost
Weeping	Occasional	Very rare
Resist eye-opening	Common	Rare
Significant injury	Rare	Common
Injury to others	Common	Rare
Tongue bite	Rare — tip of tongue	Common — lateral aspect
Incontinence	Occasional	Common
Confusion	Rare	Common

Adapted from Smith[5] and Mellers.[9]

abrupt recovery. Episodic motionless unresponsiveness for >5 minutes is highly suspicious of a nonepileptic attack disorder.[8] Table 2.3 outlines useful differences in differentiating epilepsy from psychogenic nonepileptic attacks.

Sleep Disorders

Sleep disorders commonly accompany epilepsy; obstructive sleep apnea appears twice as commonly in people with epilepsy compared to the background population. There are three main categories of sleep disorders.

1. Sleep-wake cycle disorders.
2. Parasomnias or sleep-intrusive behavior.
3. Sleep disorders associated with medical or psychiatric illness.

Parasomnias are commonly misdiagnosed as epilepsy; conversely, nocturnal seizures are commonly mistaken for sleep disorders. The main distinguishing clue is the timing of events: sleep disorders tend to occur during specific sleep phases and at certain times of the night, whereas epilepsy in sleep occurs from any sleep phase. The distinction is essentially clinical and even with polysomnography, sleep latency testing and video EEG, often remains difficult.

Sleep Disorders Misdiagnosed as Epilepsy

Several sleep syndromes cause confusion with epilepsy:

- *Narcolepsy* is a disorder of rapid eye movement (REM) sleep. The full syndrome is characterized by sleep attacks, cataplexy, sleep paralysis, and hypnagogic (prior to falling asleep) or hypnopompic hallucinations.
- *Sleep attacks* manifest as uncontrollable urges to sleep, notably at inappropriate times, e.g., during meals or conversations.
- *Cataplexy* is characterized by a sudden loss of muscle tone with emotional stimuli, e.g., laughter, noise, surprise, or anger. There is no alteration of consciousness.
- *Sleep paralysis* usually occurs on wakening and comprises feeling awake but being unable to move. This is often very frightening and is often associated with symptoms of panic.
- *Obstructive sleep apnea* is common, especially in overweight men with large neck sizes who develop upper airway collapse during sleep leading to loud snoring, frequent apneic spells in sleep, morning headache, and marked sleep fragmentation causing daytime somnolence. The sleep attacks and the daytime somnolence both can be confused with epilepsy. Furthermore, the resulting sleep deprivation may exacerbate pre-existing epilepsy.
- *Restless legs and periodic limb movements in sleep*. Restless legs syndrome is characterized by an unpleasant sensation in the legs, with an overwhelming urge to move the legs. It is usually worse in the evenings and at night. It is associated with periodic limb movements in sleep—brief repetitive jerks of the legs every 20-40 seconds causing frequent arousals—which can easily be misdiagnosed as frontal lobe epilepsy.
- *Sleep-wake transition disorders*, e.g., benign hypnic or myoclonic jerks, occur on falling to sleep.
- *Nocturnal enuresis*, common in children and possibly occurring in the elderly, often raises suspicion of nocturnal epilepsy.
- *Non-REM parasomnias* include sleepwalking, night terrors, and confusional arousal. Individuals are usually confused during the event and amnesic afterwards.
- *REM parasmonias* are nightmares during REM sleep, often associated with drugs (L-dopa compounds) and neurological and psychological disease.
- *REM sleep behavioral disorder* results from loss of the normal motor inhibition of REM sleep, typically in Parkinson's disease and multiple systems atrophy, causing patients to "act out" their dreams. It is often exacerbated by L-dopa medications.

Epilepsy Misdiagnosed as Sleep Disorder

Autosomal dominant nocturnal frontal lobe epilepsy was recently recognized as a familial epilepsy; many cases had probably been previously misdiagnosed as a sleep disorder (the syndrome was sometimes formerly labeled as paroxysmal nocturnal dystonia). Patients develop clusters of nocturnal brief motor seizures, often complex and violent and usually with retained consciousness.[10,11] The surface EEG sometimes even remains normal during seizures owing to the epileptogenic zone being relatively deep in the supplementary motor area.

Investigation of Blackouts

Blackouts are diagnosed clinically, but some investigations can support the diagnosis, identify the underlying cause, and clarify the epilepsy syndrome diagnosis. However, investigations rarely substitute for an accurate history and eye-witnessed account.

Electrocardiogram (ECG)

ECG is the most important initial investigation. Although the interictal ECG is normal in patients with epilepsy, and no particular ECG features predict propensity to SUDEP, its value is to identify or exclude epilepsy mimics, e.g., long QT syndrome, hypertrophic cardiomyopathy. These conditions, though rare, are potentially preventable causes of sudden death. Furthermore, specialized cardiology tests may then be indicated, e.g., head-up tilt-table testing, echocardiography, and prolonged heart rate monitoring.

Electroencephalography (EEG)

Electroencephalography, initially developed in the early 20th century, analyzes small electrical changes produced by the superficial cerebral cortex, measured by using scalp electrodes. Patients and doctors often wrongly regard EEG as a diagnostic test for epilepsy and a routine investigation for blackouts. However, unless an actual seizure is captured on the recording, an EEG can only support a clinical diagnosis of epilepsy.

"Epileptiform" activity on an EEG does not necessarily mean that the diagnosis is epilepsy; 0.5-3% of the healthy population have an abnormal EEG.[12] Epileptiform activity without epilepsy may accompany brain tumors, severe intellectual disability, congenital brain injury, and may follow brain surgery. Conversely, the EEG is often normal in people with epilepsy. Even during seizures, surface EEG is may not capture abnormal electrical discharges (rarely) if the epileptic focus is buried deeply within the cerebral cortex.

Therefore an EEG must only be interpreted in the correct clinical context; a full description of the attacks is essential to the EEG reporter. A routine baseline, interictal EEG lasts 20–30 minutes and involves recording during wakefulness (including a period of hyperventilation and of photic stimulation). Video recording of the procedure is helpful, because it provides a visual record of any events. Recording soon after the last seizure can increase the EEG yield further, as can repeating the awake recording, recording during sleep following prior sleep deprivation, or making more prolonged recordings over days.

Common EEG Indications

- To support a clinical diagnosis of epilepsy.
- To aid epilepsy syndrome diagnosis (some syndromes have characteristic EEG findings).
- To demonstrate photosensitivity (5% of epilepsy patients).
- To demonstrate postictal discharge slowing (useful in distinguishing epilepsy from nonepileptic attacks).
- To provoke nonepileptic attacks (these commonly occur during photic stimulation).
- To diagnose and manage convulsive and nonconvulsive status epilepticus.

Prolonged EEG monitoring, video telemetry, and ambulatory monitoring are useful for frequent undiagnosed blackouts, especially nonepileptic attack disorders, sleep disorders, and in the intellectually disabled, for whom a good description of their attacks is lacking. These recordings also provide information on patients with established epilepsy to determine the seizure type and the amount of epileptiform activity, to identify additional nonepileptic attacks, to study any precipitants, and to localize the epileptic focus in potentially surgical cases. More invasive depth EEG electrodes are useful in planning therapeutic surgical interventions for patients with focal epilepsy.

Brain Imaging

Computed Tomography (CT)

Computed tomography (CT) scanning is readily available and can provide information on brain symmetry and on large potentially epileptogenic lesions like infarction or tumors. It is particularly useful where there are calcified abnormalities and skull changes. However, CT is insufficiently sensitive to use as definitive imaging in most patients with epilepsy.

Magnetic Resonance Imaging (MRI)

MRI has essentially replaced CT as the imaging of choice for epilepsy because of its sensitivity and specificity in identifying the etiology of epilepsy. However, MRI is not widely available, making CT sometimes still the appropriate initial investigation. The more commonly identified abnormalities on MRI are hippocampal sclerosis, cortical malformations, and benign cortical tumors (ganglioglioma and dysembryoplastic neuroepithelial tumor). Functional MRI and MR spectroscopy can add additional information, sometimes identifying potentially resectable focal abnormalities in MRI-negative patients.

MRI Indications

Clinical best practice is to obtain MRI in all adults presenting with epilepsy, apart from those with definite idiopathic generalized epilepsy. Table 2.4 outlines specific indications for MRI in patients with epilepsy. Figures 2.3A and 2.3B show the MRI scan appearances of hippocampal sclerosis and of a cavernous hemangioma (cavernoma).

Table 2.4 MRI Indications in epilespy

Partial seizures, with or without secondary generalization, with onset at any age
Epilepsy with onset in first year of life or beyond aged 20 years.
Focal neurological signs.
Focal EEG abnormalities.
Loss of seizure control.
Change in seizure pattern and type.
Epilepsy refractory to first-line medication.

Adapted from Berkovic et al.[13]

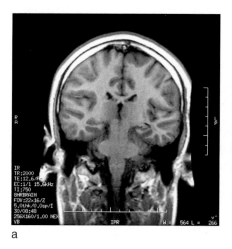 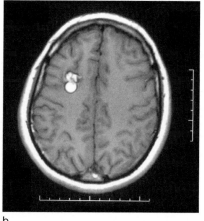

a   b

Fig. 2.3 (A) MRI brain scan showing left-sided hippocampal sclerosis. (B) MRI scan showing right-sided frontal lobe cavernoma

Management

The management of epilepsy and the choice of antiepileptic medication are considered in detail in Chapters 6 and 7. Here we consider some general and lifestyle aspects which need to be addressed as part of epilepsy management.

Living with Epilepsy

Improving patients' understanding and knowledge about their chronic conditions can potentially improve their medication concordance and facilitate the doctor-patient relationship.

For most adults with epilepsy, and especially those with intellectual disability, the condition is lifelong; as with all chronic illnesses, epilepsy becomes part of their daily lives. Individuals living with epilepsy often have concerns other than diagnosis and management, especially regarding epilepsy's impact upon day-to-day life, including family life, children, schooling, education, career, insurance, driving, alcohol, and "flashing lights."

Many people erroneously believe that people with epilepsy must have severe lifestyle restrictions imposed upon them. However, apart from driving, most people with epilepsy can and should live a full and active life. Sensible advice might include avoiding obvious provoking factors, e.g., sleep deprivation, excess alcohol, and illicit drugs. People with epilepsy can generally be encouraged to participate in leisure activities and sports, particularly team sports; common sense can determine which activities are suitable. However, special care may be needed for certain potentially dangerous situations, e.g., bathing alone, swimming, and isolated sports such as sailing and hill walking.

Driving

Drivers with epilepsy have a greater risk of accidents and road death.[14] Decisions on driving eligibility in the UK are made by the Driving and Vehicle Licensing Agency (DVLA).

Epilepsy

- **Group 1 licenses** (motorcars and motorcycles) require seizure freedom for 12 months, or if the seizures are solely sleep-related, then this pattern must have been established for 3 years prior to obtaining a license.

- **Group 2 licenses** (trucks >3.5 tons, passenger vehicles of 9+ seats, and vehicles for hire) require seizure freedom and freedom from antiepileptic medication for 10 years.

Single seizure: The same DVLA regulations for Group 1 licenses apply.
Provoked seizures: the regulation depends upon the cause:

- Those related to transient events, e.g., anesthesia, are dealt with individually by the DVLA.
- Those provoked by alcohol and illicit drugs require 1-year seizure free (Group 1).

Changing Medication

When seizure-free drivers taper or change medication (Group 1), they are advised to refrain from driving from the time of starting the change until six months following completion of the change.

Specific rules apply for brain tumor, subarachnoid hemorrhage, head injury, and neurosurgery.

Thus in the UK, the DVLA makes the driving eligibility decision, and not the patient's clinician. The DVLA's "At a glance" guide is updated every six months at www.**dvla**.gov.uk.

Photosensitivity

The media and television and film industry often portray epilepsy as a photosensitive condition, which heightens concern about the safety of computers and video entertainments in people with epilepsy. However, only 5% of people with epilepsy actually are photosensitive, with onset usually in childhood but maximal in teenage years; almost invariably it indicates an idiopathic generalized epilepsy. Photosensitivity can be easily diagnosed with EEG photic stimulation using alternating light strobe frequencies, so allowing patients to be easily identified and informed. For the vast majority of people with epilepsy there is no increased seizure risk when exposed to televisions, computer games, and flashing disco lights. However, for individuals who are photosensitive, it is reasonable to advise viewing television at a reasonable distance, in a well-lit room, and using the remote control to change channels.

Neuropsychology

Used together with the clinical history and other investigations, neuropsychology is helpful in the diagnosis and management of epilepsy. Neuropsychology identifies and quantifies cognitive function in terms of intelligence, language, memory, perception, and executive function. In patients with epilepsy, neuropsychologists can aid diagnosis, evaluate medication effects, monitor cognitive decline, and make key observations in pre- and postoperative surgical evaluations. Neuropsychologists can also help the assessment of nonepileptic attack disorders, eliciting precipitating factors and ultimately facilitating their management and continuing care.

Special Client Groups

Epilepsy is very heterogeneous: what is true for one individual may not be for the next. Age, sex, and social background each give grounds for special consideration. Special groups among patients with epilepsy include neonates, young children, teenagers, elderly, women, and the intellectually disabled.

Intellectually Disabled

Large epidemiological studies suggest that about 30% of people with intellectual disabilities (IQ < 70) have epilepsy. In general, such patients require special management owing to the severity and treatment resistance of the epilepsy itself, their often complex comorbidities, and the social, psychological, and other complex psychiatric interplays compounding the diagnostic and therapeutic consultations. Epilepsy in the learning-disabled population can be caused by congenital brain abnormalities, developmental anomalies, chromosomal abnormalities (e.g., Down syndrome, fragile-X syndrome, tuberous sclerosis, or Angelman syndrome) or can result later in life from brain damage through trauma, hemorrhage, or surgery.

Neonates

Seizures more commonly occur in neonates than at other lifetime stages, reflecting a greater seizure propensity of the immature brain. Major causes of neonatal seizures include hypoxic-ischemic encephalopathy, intracranial hemorrhage, cerebral infarction, cerebral malformations, meningitis, and metabolic abnormalities (e.g., hypoglycemia and inborn errors of metabolism). Specific epilepsy syndromes can also occur in neonates, e.g., benign idiopathic neonatal convulsions (fifth day fits), benign familial neonatal convulsions, or early myoclonic encephalopathy. However, many conditions are easily confused with epilepsy, e.g., certain motor disturbances, sleep-related movements, breath-holding attacks, and immature brainstem reflexes; great care must be taken not to misdiagnose epilepsy in this situation.[15]

Young Children

Febrile seizures are the commonest cause of seizures in young children. They are defined as seizures of cerebral origin occurring in association with a febrile illness but not involving infection of the central nervous system. Febrile seizures comprise the commonest problem in pediatric neurology, having occurred at least once in 2–4% of 5-year-olds.[16] They typically begin in the second year of life, the greatest risk being between six months and three years. The temperature is usually greater than 38°C. The seizures are usually brief, generalized, settle spontaneously and, in the vast majority, do not affect subsequent intelligence, brain function, or behavior. Overall, the risk of subsequent epilepsy is no greater than for the general population; however, a small minority with more prolonged febrile seizures can later develop complex partial seizures associated with hippocampal sclerosis.

The other important epilepsy diagnosis in young children is the benign epilepsies of childhood. The commonest is benign childhood epilepsy with centrotemporal spikes (benign Rolandic epilepsy). This typically presents between 6 and 8 years of age with simple partial seizures (usually limb shaking and drooling) arising from sleep; the interictal EEG shows characteristic centrotemporal spikes. The prognosis is excellent (hence the importance of its recognition), with almost all cases remitting by puberty. Other causes of blackouts in young children include vasovagal syncope, migraine phenomena (including benign vertigo of childhood), breath-holding attacks and, often later in childhood, nonepileptic attack disorders.

More than many other medical conditions of childhood, epilepsy generates important social and psychological issues for the individual, the parents, and caregivers. Schooling and education, peer pressure, and parental fear and anxiety are important factors to address in the overall management and well-being of the patient.

Teenagers

Teenagers typically seek independence from their parents and from the restrictions of childhood and acceptance by their peers. The transition of childhood to adulthood is stressful enough without the additional burden of a chronic disorder such as epilepsy. Important considerations in teenagers include:

- Is the diagnosis correct? (Consider nonepileptic attack disorder).
- Anxiety of individuals and their parents.
- Medication concordance.
- Education and career choices.
- Sexual choices and contraception.
- Driving.

The most important epilepsy syndrome presenting in the teenage years is JME (see above). This is important to recognize (sometimes requiring a closed question about morning jerks), because the choice of medication is limited (valproate is the most effective, but carbamazepine may worsen the myoclonus and absences). Complete seizure freedom is expected on medication, yet it is a lifelong condition requiring long-term medication (even if many years seizure free).

Elderly

The age-specific incidence of epilepsy is "U" shaped, with neonates and the elderly showing the highest rates. Most (75%) elderly-onset epilepsy is explained as being due to cerebrovascular disease[17]; other causes include tumors, dementia, and head trauma. The diagnosis is again entirely clinical, relying upon history and eye-witnessed accounts. However, such detailed descriptions may be less achievable in frail elderly people living alone. Furthermore, comorbidities such as ischemic heart disease and cognitive impairment and polypharmacy can make diagnosing epilepsy in an elderly person a considerable challenge. An epilepsy diagnosis carries immense medical and social implications for an elderly person, including risk of injury, confusion, depression, fear of isolation, and lack of independence. Furthermore, an underlying ischemic-related arrhythmogenic cardiac syncope (easily attributed to epilepsy) may easily prove fatal, yet the misdiagnosis of epilepsy may remain unrecognized even after death.

Women

Women with epilepsy justify special consideration. The choice of antiepileptic medication in women may be influenced by potential cosmetic side effects, by contraceptive issues, by hormonal influence on seizures, but most of all by the potential teratogenicity of certain antiepileptic medications.

- **Cosmetic effects** include hirustism and acne (phenytoin) and weight gain (sodium valproate).
- **Contraceptive pill**. Enzyme-inducing antiepileptic medications may allow hormonal contraceptive failure from enhanced metabolism of estrogen metabolites. Therefore women taking carbamazepine, oxcarbazepine, and phenytoin and, to a lesser extent, those taking lamotrigine, tiagabine, topiramate, or zonisamide require specific contraceptive advice and advice on additional barrier contraceptive measures.
- **Teratogenicity** is a major influence on antiepileptic prescribing in women. The incidence of major malformations following antiepileptic monotherapy exposure is 3.7%; following polytherapy it is 6%, but the greatest risk is with polytherapy combinations involving valproate at 6.2%.[18] All women planning pregnancy are recommended to take folate 5 mg daily to try to prevent neural

tube defects, although its evidence for benefit to humans fetuses exposed to antiepileptic drugs is still lacking.
- **Cyclical hormonal changes** sometimes clearly influence seizure control. Catamenial clustering of seizures around the menstrual period offers an opportunity for intermittent antiepileptic therapy.[19] Women with epilepsy generally have fewer children than those without.[20] Pregnancy, labor, and ultimately parenthood in women with epilepsy merit specific advice; throughout pregnancy women with active epilepsy should maintain regular contact with the obstetric and epilepsy services, e.g., by joint midwife and epilepsy specialist nurse clinics.

Conclusion

Epilepsy is a common, complex, and often chronic condition affecting all ages. The diagnosis of epilepsy can be surprisingly challenging, and relies not upon tests but upon a full and accurate history, including an eye-witnessed account. Its management encompasses lifestyle choices, antiepileptic drugs, surgical and psychological interventions, and requires special considerations for certain client groups. A better understanding of the cellular and genetic mechanisms underlying epilepsy and considerable progress in the production of new antiepileptic medications have changed the complexion of epilepsy, even in the past decade. The stigma of epilepsy from previous centuries is beginning to lift. People with epilepsy can now in many cases realistically expect to become seizure free without adverse medication effects. Greater clinical openness and widely available information on the Internet and elsewhere have increased knowledge and awareness about epilepsy among patients, their relatives, and the voluntary sector. People with epilepsy can now expect to be better integrated into home, working, and community life, and ultimately lead fuller, more independent, active social lives than had ever been previously possible.

Acknowledgments We thank the staff of the EEG department, Dr. Gareth Payne and Dr. Benny Thomas, University Hospital of Wales, for the EEG figures.

References

1. Commission on Classification and Terminology of the International League Against Epilepsy. (1989) Proposal for revised classification of epilepsies and epileptic syndromes. Epilepsia 30:389–399.
2. Sander JW, Shorvon SD. (1996) Epidemiology of the epilepsies. J Neurol Neurosurg Psychiatry 61:433-443.
3. Sander JW. (2003) The epidemiology of epilepsy revisited. Curr Opinion Neurol 16:166-170.
4. MacDonald BK, Cockerell OC, Sander JW, et al. (2000) The incidence and lifetime prevalence of the neurological disorders in a prospective community-based study in the UK. Brain 123:665–676.

5. Smith PEM. (2001) If it's not epilepsy .... J Neurol Neurosurg Psychiatry 70 (Suppl 2): ii9–ii14.
6. Smith D, Defalla BA, Chadwick DW. (1999) The misdiagnosis of epilepsy and the management of refractory epilepsy in a specialist clinic.Q J Med 92: 15–23.
7. Benbadis SR, Allen HW. (2000) An estimate of the prevalence of psychogenic non-epileptic seizures. Seizure 9: 280–281.
8. Meierkord H, Will B, Fish D, et al. (1991) The clinical features and prognosis of pseudoseizures diagnosed using video-EEG telemetry.Neurology 41: 1643–1646.
9. Mellers JDC. (2005)The approach to patients with 'non-epileptic seizures'. Postgrad Med J 81: 498–504.
10. Scheffer IE, Bhatia KP, Lopes-CendesI et al.(1995) Autosomal dominant nocturnal frontal lobe epilepsy — A distinct clinical syndrome. Brain 118: 61–73.
11. Scheffer IE, Bhatia KP, Lopes-Cendes I et al. (1994) Autosomal dominant nocturnal frontal lobe epilepsy misdiagnosed as a sleep disorder. Lancet 343: 515–517.
12. Gregory RP, Oates T, Merry RTG. (1993). EEG epileptiform abnormalities in candidates for aircrew training. Electroenceph Clin Neurophysiol 86: 75–77.
13. Berkovic SF, Duncan JS, Barkovich A, et al. (1997) ILAE commission neuroimaging recommendations for neuroimaging of patients with epilepsy. Epilepsia 38: 1–2.
14. Hansotia P, Broste SK. (1993). Epilepsy and traffic safety. Epilepsia 34: 852–858.
15. Levene MI, Troune JQ. (1986) Causes of neonatal convulsions. Arch Dis Child 61: 78–79.
16. Nelson KB, Ellenberg JH. (1978) Prognosis in children with febrile seizures. Pediatrics 61: 720–727.
17. Sander JW, Hart YM, Johnson AL, et al. (1990) National General Practice Study of Epilepsy: Newly diagnosed epileptic seizures in a general population. Lancet 336: 1267–1271.
18. Morrow J, Russell A, Guthrie E, et al. (2006) Malformation risks of antiepileptic drugs in pregnancy: A prospective study from the UK Epilepsy and Pregnancy Register. J Neurol Neurosurg Psychiatry 77: 193–198.
19. Duncan S, Read CL, Brodie MJ. (1993). How common is catamenial epilepsy? Epilepsia 34: 827–831.
20. Olafsson E, Hauser WA, Gudmundsson G. (1998) Fertility in patients with epilepsy: A population based study. Neurology 51: 71–73.

Chapter 3
Epidemiology of Epilepsy in Persons with Intellectual Disabilities

S. W. Brown

Introduction

The epilepsies represent one of the most significant groups of conditions that may be associated with intellectual disabilities (ID). There is a general consensus that the incidence (new cases arising in a population in a period of time) and prevalence (the number of people in a population with the diagnosis at a given point in time) of seizure disorders in people with ID are greatly increased compared to the general population, and that the spectrum of epilepsy syndromes and seizure types represented are more refractory and difficult to treat. However, such generalized statements disguise a complex and varied range of presentations, and this chapter will attempt to disentangle some of these relationships in the present state of knowledge. When interpreting the results of studies it is important to remember that not all epileptologists are specialists in the psychiatry of ID, and not all researchers who work in the ID field are epilepsy specialists. Learning disabilities and seizure disorders may be defined or classified in different ways in different studies, and there may be geographical variations in presentation for various reasons. Also, other factors, including developments in prenatal screening, obstetrics, and postnatal care, may yet have a significant impact on the epidemiology of epilepsy in the ID population.

Definitions and Variations

Learning Disability

The standard internationally accepted way of defining ID (also known as intellectual disability or mental retardation) in the *International Statistical Classification of Diseases and Related Health Problems* (ICD-10)[1] is based on two main components: low cognitive ability defined as an Intelligence Quotient (IQ) score of < 70 and diminished social competence. Onset has to be during the developmental period. Intelligence Quotient is further used to differentiate four categories of severity (mild, moderate, severe, and profound). If IQ alone were used as the criterion,

V.P. Prasher, M.P. Kerr (eds.) *Epilepsy and Intellectual Disabilities*,
DOI: 10.1007/978-1-84800-259-3_3, © Springer Science+Business Media, LLC 2008

about 3% of the population would be regarded as qualifying. This is a reflection of the way that tests are constructed.[2] The *Diagnostic and Statistical Manual of Mental Disorders-IV* (DSM-IV)[3] places some additional importance on problems with adaptive behavior in making a diagnosis.

These definitions imply that some people whose IQ is below 70 may not be regarded as having ID. In addition, some studies have included people with an IQ of <70 in prevalence studies of intellectual disability, stressing the importance of overall level of functioning and whether the person is receiving special services. In this way, for example, Beange and Taplin[4] added an extra 14 subjects to the 346 identified by IQ in their study of the adult population of Sydney, Australia. Other studies, such as that of Bhasin and colleagues,[5] have used IQ as the main or only criterion in determining prevalence.

Another way of gathering data is to study the numbers of people receiving the relevant welfare benefits or special educational or social care provision that is available for people with ID. Not surprisingly, widely varying results can be obtained in this way. The Centers for Disease Control's Morbidity & Mortality Weekly Report in 1996[6] described wide fluctuations in the reported prevalence per 1,000 population of mental retardation between different states of the United States, ranging in children from 31.4 (Alabama) to 3.2 (New Jersey) and in adults from 15.7 (Virginia) to 2.5 (Alaska). Although some real differences in prevalence might well exist, it was recommended that some effort was needed to explain these large differences, which might be consequent on social practice.

McConkey and colleagues[7] point out that differences in the demographic profiles of the underlying general populations may also have an effect, but that this has received scant attention. They also suggest that in affluent societies with national coverage of services, it is likely that "administrative" and "true" prevalence rates are probably convergent for persons with severe disabilities.

The United Kingdom (UK) Department of Health White Paper *"Valuing People"*[8] gives a figure for the number of people with a ID for England that equates to about 3% of the population. This is the same as the expected number of people who would have an IQ of less than 70, and is a consequence of the way IQ tests are constructed. If such official government figures are accurate, it raises a question about the significance of criteria other than IQ that are necessary for both ICD-10[1] and DSM-IV[3] diagnoses. If the figure of approximately 3% prevalence is applied across the UK using latest census data, this gives a figure of 1.824 million people of all ages with ID.

Results of epidemiological studies of ID thus may fluctuate for a number of reasons, not all of which may be due to real differences in incidence or prevalence.

Epilepsy

Epilepsy is usually defined as the tendency to have recurrent seizures. The lifetime risk of having at least one epileptic seizure over an 80-year life span in the United States has been estimated to be as high as 1 in 10,[9] and the lifetime risk of acquiring a diagnosis of epilepsy is said to be about 3.5%.[10]

The Joint Epilepsy Council of Great Britain and Ireland (JEC) has published a summary of a consensus view of the current epidemiology of epilepsy in the UK and Ireland.[11] Regarding prevalence, the consensus view is that the age standardized prevalence rate of epilepsy in the UK is 7.5 per 1,000, which approximates to 456,000 people in the UK based on 2003 census data. The prevalence changes with age, from 1 in 279 children (3.6 per 1,000) under 16 years of age, to 1 in 91 (11 per 1,000) for people aged over 65. The JEC document also states that more than one in five people with epilepsy have ID. Figures for annual incidence are given as overall approximately 46 per 100,000 (0.46 cases per 1,000) of population, which gives 27,400 new cases diagnosed per year in the UK, or 105 new cases each working day of the year. Other studies have shown that incidence varies with age, with peaks at each end of life. In the European White Paper on Epilepsy[12] the authors, noting that recent studies indicate an increase in incidence rates in the elderly, raise the question of whether incidence may be underestimated, which may lead to under treatment.

Overall Incidence and Prevalence of Epilepsy in the ID Population

Older institution-based studies do not greatly inform current practice, although these historical observations emphasize the extra dependency and need for support that people with ID might require if they also develop epilepsy and inform us of other significant co-existing conditions such as cerebral palsy.[13,14]

Population-based studies have been carried out more recently, and available data could reasonably apply in the developed, industrialized world. Case register studies from Camberwell[15–17] and from Aberdeen[18,19] confirm a marked increase in the prevalence of epilepsy if ID is present, with the overall prevalence remaining consistent from childhood to early adult life, since although some epilepsies of early onset improve, others begin in adolescence. The Aberdeen study also suggested postnatal injury and associated disabilities to be particular risk factors for this increased prevalence of epilepsy, and both studies showed that the rate of epilepsy was higher when ID was more severe.

Some of the most significant work has come from Scandinavian, particularly Swedish, population studies. Forsgren and colleagues,[20] in a whole population study of a Swedish county, found a point prevalence of 20% of active epilepsy in people with ID, the rate varying from 23% of those with severe ID to 11% of those where the ID was classified as mild. The proportion having daily to weekly seizures was 26.8%, with only 32% having been seizure-free for the past year, and in 27.7% the epilepsy had commenced before the age of one year.

Steffenberg and colleagues,[21,22] investigating a population of children in Göteborg aged 6–13 years, found 15% of those with mid-ID had epilepsy compared with 45% of those with more severe ID. In this study 44% of the children had daily to weekly seizures, in contrast to the findings of Forsgren, whose study population was drawn from across the lifespan. This suggests that the manifestation of epilepsy in children with ID may be more severe with greater seizure frequency than in adults. The Göteborg study was also consistent with the earlier observation from the Aberdeen cohort that associated brain damage giving rise to both ID and epilepsy was perhaps the most significant factor in seizure outcome.

Sillanpää, in a 1999 review[23] of epilepsy and ID, observed "In population-based studies, the prevalence of ID in patients who have epilepsy seems to be of the same order as epilepsy in ID." Do findings from these different sources give the same numbers for those affected in a population? Taking the UK as an example, the JEC figure of 456,000 people with epilepsy of whom one in five may have ID would predict 91,200 as the number with co-existing conditions. However, *Valuing People* gives a population prevalence of ID overall of around 3%, with 2.5% being mild/moderate and 0.5% being severe/profound. Taking the same census data for the whole UK as the JEC uses, would give an overall figure of 1,824,000 people with ID in whom 1,520,000 would be mild/moderate and 304,000 severe or profound. At first glance this is discrepant, since 20% of 1,824,000 gives 364,800 as the figure for people with both epilepsy and ID, four times greater than the previous estimate. Even if we extrapolate Forsgren's figures for epilepsy prevalence according to severity of ID, this figure only comes down to 237,120. However, if we pool all the suggested figures from the Camberwell, Aberdeen, and Göteborg studies, as Lhatoo and Sander have done,[24] the prevalence of epilepsy in mild ID may be as low as 6%, which brings the overall figure down about 150,000, which is closer to the predicted figure, though still high. The only conclusions that can reasonably be drawn from this are that epilepsy and ID occur together far more often than by chance, and that more research is needed to take into account the increasing life expectancy of the population, such that extrapolating from pediatric data is increasingly inappropriate.

A Note on Mortality

It is generally accepted that a diagnosis of epilepsy carries a risk of premature death two to three times higher than in the general population[25] and that most of these premature deaths are directly related to the epilepsy itself. At least half of the excess mortality may be due to a condition called Sudden Unexpected Death in Epilepsy (SUDEP), for which the most significant risk factor is the continued occurrence of seizures, especially generalized tonic-clonic seizures.[26] Intellectual disability is also often regarded as risk factor,[27] and one study found young people with severe epilepsy and ID had a death rate 15.9 times greater than expected.[28] Walczak, further reviewing data from his original 1998 study, stated that seizure frequency and ID are independent risk factors. [29] However, data from the UK National Sentinel Audit suggested that for those with ID who died an epilepsy-related death, it was possible that lack of contact with a specialist ID clinical team might be a risk factor. One population-based study in Cornwall, UK, supported this view,[30] with the implication that good quality treatment, career training, and especially attention to rescue medication might substantially reduce mortality. Thus the epidemiology of epilepsy-related mortality in the ID population might be altered by certain management approaches. In the absence of such approaches, however, there is a potential for substantially increased epilepsy-related mortality in the ID population.

A Note on Concomitant Psychiatric Disorder

It is often stated that epilepsy, especially chronic epilepsy, carries a risk of associated psychiatric disorder. This is particularly true for the association with psychosis, which according to Krishnamoorthy[31] is 10 times greater than in the general population. Quite separately, people with ID are said to have higher rates of mental health problems than the rest of the population, often stated as three to five times greater than expected, with some studies showing very significantly greater risk for schizophrenia.[32] As Krishnamoorthy noted in a further review,[33] the literature on psychopathology among subjects with epilepsy and ID is sparse and contradictory. Nevertheless, Scandinavian population-based studies once again give the clearest picture. In the Göteborg children's study it was found that 59% of those with ID and active epilepsy had at least one psychiatric diagnosis, including 38% with autism spectrum disorders. The authors felt that these observed figures were possibly lower than the actual prevalence because some children lacked the skills and mobility to exhibit behavioral and emotional problems that might lead to diagnosis.[34] Lund, reporting a population-based study of adults,[35-36] found that among the ID population psychiatric disorders were strongly correlated with epilepsy, with 59% of those with both ID and epilepsy having a psychiatric disorder compared to 26% of those with ID but no epilepsy. This study was carried out in the early 1980s, and it is possible that such figures may change as the age distribution of the population changes, emphasizing the need for more up-to-date research.

Some Syndromes of Developmental Disability Related to Epilepsy

Cerebral Palsy

Cerebral palsy is a chronic nonprogressive cerebral disorder in young children that results in impaired motor function.[37] As people with the condition live longer into adulthood, anecdotal observations suggest that the "nonprogressive" part of the definition may require qualification. Cerebral palsy is also broadly subdivided into four types: hemiplegic, diplegic, tetraplegic, and dystonic. The rates of epilepsy occurring in these different types has been reviewed by Aicardi.[38]

Hemiplegic cerebral palsy is typically associated with damage in the area supplied by the middle cerebral artery, and the clinical features become obvious within the first few months of life. Epilepsies occur in 34–60%, and tend to be partial, arising from scar tissue around the damaged area. The middle cerebral artery supplies the lateral cortex of the frontal, parietal, and temporal lobes, including the sensorimotor cortex, but not the occipital or inferior temporal cortex, which are supplied by the posterior cerebral artery, and the resultant localization-related epilepsy reflects the distribution of the artery concerned.

Diplegic cerebral palsy has a high correlation with very-low-birth-weight survivors. The cerebral insult is prenatal and typically subcortical, so that the rate of epilepsy is relatively low. If the insult is especially severe, there may be cortical involvement leading to a partial or generalized epilepsy, which is seen in 16–27%. In tetraplegic cerebral palsy there is widespread cortical involvement which can lead to multi-focal or symptomatic generalized epilepsies in 50–90% of cases. Dystonic cerebral palsy arises from basal ganglia damage or mal-development, and since the cortex is relatively spared, epilepsy is not inevitable. Seizure disorders arise in 23–26%, the occurrence of epilepsy suggests global cortical involvement in these cases, and the presentation is therefore usually a symptomatic generalized epilepsy.

By no means all people with cerebral palsy have ID. Much research has been carried out on children and young people, with relatively fewer available data for adults. In the Rochester, Minnesota, study, Kudrjavcec and colleagues[39] found the cumulative risk of epilepsy in people with cerebral palsy to be 33% by age 16 years, and in the Aberdeen study, Goulden and colleague noted that when cerebral palsy and ID occurred together the cumulative risk of epilepsy was 38% by age 22 years. Delgado and colleagues[40] showed that epilepsy in this context was particularly refractory, with only 13% showing a two-year remission, although this seemed to be more related to the cerebral palsy than to the ID. It seems that the presence of ID makes epilepsy slightly more likely to occur where there is cerebral palsy, perhaps a consequence of the overall severity of the cerebral insult. Where there is ID, the presence of cerebral palsy seems to add more to the risk of developing epilepsy. Corbett and colleagues[41] in an early study found that in a population with ID the risk of epilepsy was three times higher if cerebral palsy was also present. Some interesting findings from an Italian study by Arpino and colleagues[42] included observations that there was an increased family history of epilepsy in first-degree relatives of people with ID and cerebral palsy, and that the combination of cerebral palsy, ID, and epilepsy was less likely where the mother was less than 32 years old when the child was born, and also less likely to be associated with premature birth or low birth weight. D'Amelio and colleagues[43] speculate that of the cerebral insults leading to cerebral palsy, those associated with low birth weight or prematurity are different to those that occur in full-term babies, and that the latter may be more likely to develop subsequent epilepsy, in addition to the contribution of a positive family history of epilepsy.

There is a paucity of long-term follow-up studies, and little information regarding the prognosis of cerebral palsy, let alone associated epilepsy, in later life. One primary care based study in North America reported declining rates of epilepsy in older people with cerebral palsy, with or without associated learning disability.[44] It is not clear, however, whether this represents an underlying premature mortality or a tendency in some cases to remission.

Fragile X

Fragile X syndrome is one of the most common genetic causes of ID with an approximate incidence in males of between 1 in 1,500[45] and 1 in 6,000.[46] Females are also affected, but the phenotype is more severe in males. Up to 1 in 1,000 females may be carriers. The presence of epilepsy is not influenced by the degree of ID that may be present. Most epilepsy starts before the age of 15[47] and often remits in adolescence. Musumeci and colleagues[48] found only 25% continue to have seizures in adult life. The epilepsy is usually relatively mild and responsive to treatment (although a minority may have more severe refractory seizures) and is usually described as displaying complex partial seizures (89.3% in Musumeci's study) and tonic clonic seizures (46.4%). The appearance of relatively mild epilepsy with partial onset seizures that remit in adolescence bears comparison with the epilepsy syndrome of Benign Rolandic Epilepsy, but to date genetic studies have failed to identify any obvious link between these conditions, and the similarities may be fortuitous.[49]

Rett Syndrome

Rett syndrome is a genetically determined pervasive developmental disorder with marked autistic features associated with regression that is almost exclusively seen in females. It has been estimated to occur in at least 1 in 10,000 girls,[50] though this may be an underestimate. An abnormal electroencephalogram with generalized slowing and rhythmic slow activity and epileptic-form activity such as focal and generalized spikes and sharp waves is typically seen even without clinical seizures being apparent. About half develop epilepsy. Seizure types include tonic-clonic, absence, myoclonic and atonic events as well as partial seizures, and the picture is often that of a symptomatic generalized epilepsy. Most seizures start between three and five years of age, and are described as more severe at the onset, with some improvement with age; often remission occurs in the teenage years or 20s, though this is not inevitable. The epilepsy in Rett syndrome can be difficult to treat and often responds poorly to standard antiepileptic drugs.

Disorders of Chromosome Region 15q11–q13

This interesting and relatively unstable chromosome region is associated with Angelman syndrome, Prader-Willi syndrome, and a variety of other presentations, most notably the recently described inv dup(15) syndrome. All have different phenotypes and have different associations with epilepsy.

Angelman syndrome is a result of maternal deletion of, or paternal uniparental disomy of, 15q11–q13. It is said to occur between 1 in 10,000 and 30,000 live births.[51]

More than 80% of affected individuals develop a seizure disorder, usually with onset before the age of three, and commonly presenting with a febrile convulsion.[52] The overall picture usually resembles a symptomatic generalized epilepsy with myoclonus and drop attacks predominating, but also frequent atypical absences and tonic-clonic seizures. Complex partial seizures with eye deviation and vomiting have been described. Guerrini and colleagues[52] have noted the particular presentation of the myoclonus in Angelman syndrome that can give rise to apparent long-lasting tremor. Nonconvulsive (atypical absence) status epilepticus has been described in up to 50%, and the picture often resembles Lennox-Gastaut syndrome in adulthood.[54]

Prader-Willi syndrome arises from paternal deletion of, or maternal disomy of, 15q11–q13. The characteristic physical and behavioral phenotype is well-known and includes hyperphagia. The presentation is quite unlike Angelman syndrome. There is, however, an increased rate of febrile convulsions which is shared with Angelman syndrome, and seizure disorders seem to occur in 28–46% of individuals. This is probably higher than would be expected from the degree of learning disability alone, but no distinct epilepsy phenotype has emerged.[55] There is a suggestion that seizure disorders may be more prominent in childhood and adolescence. Butler and colleagues[56] draw attention to a large number of unexplained episodes of collapse and inattention that may confuse the diagnosis, and postulate that this might be a manifestation of cataplexy. The presence of hyperphagia and epilepsy has caused some speculation as to whether topiramate may be a suitable antiepileptic drug for people with Prader-Willi syndrome, as this is known to sometimes cause appetite suppression. There are published reports on the possible beneficial effects of topiramate on self-injurious behavior in Prader-Willi syndrome,[57] with mixed reports of the effect on appetite.[58,59]

The recently described condition[60] caused by tetrasomy of 15p, together with partial tetrasomy of 15q, and known as inv dup(15), presents with autistic-like features, hypotonia, and reftactory generalized epilepsy. It bears some semblance to Angelman syndrome. The rate of epilepsy is high, although there are not yet large enough series to provide incidence or prevalence data. Onset of seizures varies from six months to nine years, the earlier onset sometimes being with infantile spasms. There are some features suggestive of Lennox-Gastaut syndrome, and refractory myoclonus may occur. The EEG shows some features of symptomatic generalized epilepsy, together with diminution or absence of some of the normal posterior brain rhythms. Seizure activity may disrupt sleep structure.

Tuberous Sclerosis

Tuberous sclerosis (TS) is a disorder causing lesions in skin and brain, as well as other organs, and may be inherited as an autosomal dominant condition with variable penetrance, although many cases (perhaps more than half) may arise from spontaneous mutations. Ahlsén and colleagues[61] found a minimum prevalence in adolescents of 1 in 6,800, which was regarded as a probable underestimate, and also suggested that at least half of all cases presenting in early childhood with severe symptoms are inherited. At least 50% of people with TS have ID; one study found this to be as high as 80%.[62] The degree of ID varies from mild to severe. There is a particularly strong association with epilepsy and with autism. Indeed Gillberg[63] suggests that where ID, epilepsy, and autism coexist, this should serve as a clinical warning that the underlying cause might be TS. About one-third of children with TS develop infantile spasms (West syndrome), and in turn may account for 25% or more of all cases of West syndrome. More than 80% develop epilepsy at some stage. Tonic-clonic and complex partial seizures are well described.[64] The type of epilepsy seen is mainly influenced by the contribution of the various brain lesions, and therefore often presents as a symptomatic localization-related or multifocal epilepsy, although a symptomatic generalized epilepsy is sometimes seen. Where epilepsy seems to be associated with a single cortical tuber or otherwise identifiable epileptogenic region, surgical treatment has claimed some success in a small number of cases studied.[65] Recently a pattern of expression of proteins related to multiple drug resistance has been described in people with TS,[66] which would not only account for some of the refractoriness to treatment that has been seen but also may have implications for using higher doses of antiepileptic drugs in this group than previously.

Down Syndrome

Down syndrome (DS) (trisomy 21) occurs in about 1 in 800 births. Epilepsy is a frequent accompaniment. About 1% of children with DS develop West syndrome (infantile spasms)[67] against a general population rate of about one in 2000,[68] although the response to treatment is often relatively good. Epilepsy in younger people with DS shows a high rate of reflex seizures such as those precipitated by noise or touch and also of the idiopathic type of generalized epilepsies with typical absences and other generalized seizure types, often with a degree of photosensitivity.[69] There are reasons why the brains of people with DS may be especially susceptible to these seizure types, with a defect in inhibitory mechanisms.[70] The prevalence of focal (localization-related) epilepsies in adolescence seems to be only slightly higher than in the general population. There does seem to be a biphasic presentation of seizure disorders in DS, Pueschel and colleagues[71] found that in 40% of people with DS who had epilepsy, the epilepsy had started in the first year of life, while a further 40% had onset after age 40 years. The prevalence of epilepsy in DS increases with age, especially for myoclonic and often other generalized seizures along with early-onset dementia of the Alzheimer type, so that in older people with DS the prevalence of epilepsy is in the region of 70–80%.[72,73] The later onset epilepsy is characterized by myoclonus as well as other generalized seizure types and has been referred to as "senile myoclonic epilepsy[74,75]." Therefore, most of the epilepsies seen in DS are of symptomatic generalized type, with absences, myoclonus, and tonic-clonic seizures predominating; reflex seizures are common.

Some Epilepsy Syndromes Related to ID

As described in the previous section, the types of epilepsy that are especially associated with ID syndromes tend to be generalized, with myoclonus, atypical absences, and drop attacks as well as tonic-clonic and some types of complex partial seizures. Of course the same epilepsy syndromes that occur in the general population are also seen in the ID population, including mesial temporal lobe epilepsy and idiopathic generalized epilepsies such as childhood absence epilepsy and juvenile myoclonic epilepsy, but there is no evidence that these are especially overrepresented in the ID population. The excess prevalence of epilepsy is largely due to symptomatic and cryptogenic generalized epilepsies of which the Lennox-Gastaut syndrome is a particular example, together with multifocal epilepsies and epilepsies that are difficult to classify. Included among the latter are the rare but interesting Landau-Kleffner syndrome (aquired epilepstic aphasia) and the related syndrome of electrical status epilepticus during slow sleep (ESES). The incidence and prevalence of both these conditions is basically unknown. Although considered rare, it is not clear to what extent undiagnosed ESES plays a part in disintegrative autistic conditions, and further epidemiological research may clarify this.

The Lennox-Gastaut syndrome is a catastrophic epilepsy of childhood, and is defined by the presence of tonic axial, atonic, and atypical absence seizures (though other seizure types typically occur), with an electroencephalogram showing slow spike-wave and a slowing or decline in intellectual development. The age of onset varies but usually lies between two and six years, and may be preceded by a history of infantile spasms (West syndrome). Symptomatic cases account for 70–78% of presentations.[76] It is rare in the overall population, accounting probably for only about 2–5% of all epilepsies, but in children with profound ID, unequivocal Lennox-Gastaut syndrome has been reported in up to 17%,[77] and in a residential special school for children with epilepsy, two-thirds were found to fulfil the diagnostic criteria for Lennox-Gastaut syndrome.[78]

Conclusions: Looking to the Future

Epilepsy occurs in people with ID more often than in people without ID. The types of epilepsy that contribute to the excess presentation include particular seizure types such as atypical absences, myoclonic seizures, tonic and atonic seizures, as well as partial onset and tonic-clonic seizures. The epilepsies associated with ID may be difficult to treat and present particular therapeutic challenges. Some genetic syndromes that give rise to ID exhibit particular epilepsy phenotypes. Currently accepted figures for incidence and prevalence of seizure disorders in relation to these syndromes, and in relation to ID overall may need to be adjusted to take into account the increasing longevity of the ID population, and also the impact of genetic screening, improved maternal nutrition during pregnancy, and improvements in perinatal care.

References

1. Internationl Statistical Classification of Disease and Related Health Problems. Tenth Revision. (1992) Geneva World Health Organization.
2. American Psychiatric Association. (1994) Diagnostic and Statistical Manual of Mental Disorders, Fourth Edition. Washington, DC, American Psychiatric Association.
3. BrownSW(2003) Towards definitions: Learning disability, mental handicap and intelligence. In Trimble MR (ed) Learning disability and epilepsy: An integrative approach. Clarius Press, London, pp. 1-16.
4. Beange OH, Taplin JE. (1996) Prevalence of intellectual disability in northern Sydney adults. J Intellect Disabil Res 40: 191-7.
5. Bhasin TK, Brocksen S, Avchen RN et al. (2006) Prevalence of four developmental disabilities among children aged 8 years — Metropolitan Atlanta Developmental Disabilities Surveillance Program, 1996 and 2000.MMWR — Morbidity & Mortality Weekly Report.55 (SS-1):1-9.
6. Anonymous. (1996) State-specific rates of mental retardation—United States, 1993. MMWR — Morbidity & Mortality Weekly Report. 45: 61–5.
7. McConkey R, Mulvany F, Barron S. (2006) Adult persons with intellectual disabilities on the island of Ireland. J Intellect Disabil Res. 50: 227–36.
8. Valuing people: A new strategy for learning disability for the 21st century. (2001) London, The Stationery Office.
9. Hauser WA, Hesdorffer DC. (1990) Epilepsy: Frequency, causes and consequences. Demos Press. New York:
10. Hauser WA, Kurland LT. (1975) The epidemiology of epilepsy in Rochester Minnesota 1935 through 1967. Epilepsia 16: 1–66.
11. Joint Epilepsy Council. (2005) Epilepsy prevalence, incidence and other statistics. Joint Epilepsy Council, Leeds.
12. EUCARE. (2003) European White Paper on Epilepsy. Epilepsia. 44 Suppl 6: 1–88.
13. Illingworth RS. (1959) Convulsions in mentally retarded children with or without cerebral palsy. J Ment Defic Res. 3: 88–93
14. Iavanainen M. (1974) A study of origins of mental retardation, Heinemann London.
15. Corbett JA. (1979) Epilepsy and the electroencephalogram in early childhood psychoses. In: Wing JK (ed), Handbook of Psychiatry, Vol. 3. Cambridge University Press. Cambridge:
16. Corbett JA. (1988) Epilepsy and mental handicap. In: Laidlaw J, Richens A, Oxley J (eds) .A textbook of epilepsy, 3rd ed. Churchill Livingstone, Edinburgh: 533–8.
17. Corbett JA. (1983) Epilepsy and mental retardation. In: Parsonage M (ed). Proceedings of the 6th International Symposium on Epilepsy, Raven Press, London. New York, 207–14.
18. Richardson SA, Koller H, Katz M et al. (1981) A functional classification of seizures and its distribution in a mentally retarded population. Am J Ment Defic 815: 457–66.
19. Goulden KJ, Shinnar S, Koller H, et al. (1991) Epilepsy in children with mental retardation: A cohort study. Epilepsia 32: 690–7.
20. Forsgren L, Edvinsson SO, Blomquist HK, et al. (1990) Epilepsy in a population of mentally retarded children and adults. Epilepsy Res 6: 234–48.
21. Steffenburg U, Hagberg G, Viggedal G, et al. (1995) Active epilepsy in mentally retarded children. I. Prevalence and additional neuro-impairments. Acta Paediatrica 84: 1147–52.
22. Steffenburg U, Hagberg G, Kyllerman M (1996) Characteristics of seizures in a population-based series of mentally retarded children with active epilepsy. Epilepsia 37: 850–6.
23. Sillanpää M. (1999) Definitions and epidemiology. In: Sillanpää M, Gram L, Johannessen SI, Tomson T (eds). Epilepsy and mental retardation. UK, Wrightson Biomedical Publishing, Petersfield, Hampshire, 1–6.
24. Lhatoo SD, Sander JWAS. (2001) The epidemiology of epilepsy and learning disability. Epilepsia. 42 (Suppl 1): 6–9.

25. Cockerell OC, Johnson A, Sander JWAS, et al. (1994) Mortality from epilepsy: Results from a prospective population-based study. Lancet 344: 918–21.
26. Hanna N J, Black M, Sander JWS, et al. (2002) The National Sentinel Clinical Audit of Epilepsy-Related Death: Epilepsy—death in the shadows. The Stationery Office. London,
27. Walczak TS, Hauser WA, Leppik IE, et al. (1998) Incidence and risk factors for sudden unexpected death in epilepsy: A prospective cohort study. Neurology 50 [Suppl 4]: 443–4.
28. Nashef L, Fish DR, Garner S et al. (1995) Sudden death in epilepsy: A study of incidence in a young cohort with epilepsy and learning disability. Epilepsia 36: 1187–94.
29. Walczak T. (2002) Sudden unexpected death in epilepsy: An update. In: Devinsky O, Westbrook LE (eds). Epilepsy and developmental disabilities, Butterworth Heinemann, Boston: 41–7.
30. Brown S, Sullivan H, Hooper M (2004) Reduction of epilepsy-related mortality in a population with intellectual disability (ID). J Intellect Disabil Res 48: 340.
31. Krishnamoorthy ES. (2002) Neuropsychiatric disorders in epilepsy: Epidemiology and classification. In: Trimble MR, Schmitz EB (eds). The neuropsychiatry of epilepsy. Cambridge University Press, Cambridge, UK: 5–17.
32. Kerker BD. Owens PL. Zigler E. et al. (2004) Mental health disorders among individuals with mental retardation: Challenges to accurate prevalence estimates. Public Health Reports 119: 409–17.
33. Krishnamoorthy ES. (2003) Neuropsychiatric epidemiology at the interface between learning disability and epilepsy. In: Trimble MR (ed). Learning disability and epilepsy: An integrative approach. Clarius Press, London: 17–26.
34. Steffenburg S, Gillberg C, Steffenburg U. (1996) Psychiatric disorders in children and adolescents with mental retardation and active epilepsy.Arch Neurol 53: 904–12.
35. Lund J. (1985) Epilepsy and psychiatric disorder in mentally retarded adults. Acta Psychiatrica Scandinavica 72: 557–62.
36. Lund J. (1985) The prevalence of psychiatric morbidity in mentally retarded adults.Acta Psychiatrica Scandinavica 72: 563–70.
37. Bax MCO. (1964) Terminology and classification of cerebral palsy. Dev Med Child Neurology 6: 295–7.
38. Aicardi J (1990) Epilepsy in brain-injured children. Dev Med Child Neurol 32: 191–202.
39. Kudrjavcev T, Schoenberg BS, Kurland LT, et al. (1985) Cerebral palsy: Survival rates, associated handicaps, and distribution by clinical subtype (Rochester, MN, 1950–1976). Neurology 35: 900–3.
40. Delgado MR, Riela AR, Mills J, et al. (1996) Discontinuation of antiepileptic drug treatment after two seizure-free years in children with cerebral palsy. Pediatrics 97: 192–197.
41. Corbett JA, Harris R, Robinson R. (1975) Epilepsy. In: Wortis J (ed). Mental retardation and developmental disabilities, Vol VII. Raven Press, New York: 79–111.
42. Arpino C, Curatolo P, Stazi MA, et al. (1999) Differing risk factors for cerebral palsy in the presence of mental retardation and epilepsy. J Child Neurol 14: 151–5.
43. D'Amelio M, Shinnar S, Hauser WA (2002) Epilepsy in children with mental retardation and cerebral palsy. In: Devinsky O, Westbrook LE (eds). Epilepsy and developmental disabilities. Butterworth-Heinemann,Woburn, MA: 3–16.
44. McDermott S, Moran R, Platt T, et al. (2005) Prevalence of epilepsy in adults with mental retardation and related disabilities in primary care. Am J Ment Retard 110: 48–56.
45. Webb TP, Bundey SE, Thake AI, et al. (1986) Population incidence and segregation ratios in the Martin-Bell syndrome. Am J Med Genet 23: 573–80.
46. Vries BB, de Ouweland AM, van den Mohkamsing S et al. (1997) Screening and diagnosis for the fragile X syndrome among the mentally retarded: An epidemiological and psychological survey. Collaborative Fragile X Study Group. Am J Human Genetics 61: 660–7.
47. Wisniewski KE, Segan SM, Miezejeski CM, et al. (1991) The Fra(X) syndrome: Neurological, electrophysiological, and neuropathological abnormalities. Am J Med Genet 38: 476–80.
48. Musumeci SA, Hagerman RJ, Ferri R, et al. (1999) Epilepsy and EEG findings in males with fragile X syndrome. Epilepsia 40: 1092–1099.

49. Gobbi G, Genton P, Pini A, et al. (2005) Epilepsies and chromosomal disorders. In: Roger J, Bureau M, Dravet C et al. (eds). Epileptic syndromes in infancy childhood and adolescence, 4th ed., John Libbey & Co Ltd., Eastleigh, UK: 467–92.

50. Hagberg B (ed). (1993) Rett Syndrome — Clinical & Biological Aspects. McKeith Press. London:

51. Stafstrom. CE (1999) Mechanism of epilepsy in mental retardation: Insights from Angelman syndrome, Down syndrome and fragile X syndrome. In: Sillanpää M, Gram L, Johannessen SI, Tomson T (eds). Epilepsy and mental retardation.Wrightson Biomedical Publishing, Petersfield, Hampshire, UK: 7–41.

52. Matsumoto A, Kumagai T, Miura K et al. (1992) Epilepsy in Angelman syndrome associated with chromosome 15q deletion. Epilepsia 33: 1083–1090.

53. Guerrini R, Lorey TM, De Bonanni P, et al. (1996) Cortical myoclonus in Angelman syndrome. Ann Neurol 40: 39–48.

54. Minassian BA, DeLorey TM, Olsen RW, et al. (1998) Angelman syndrome: Correlations between epilepsy phenotypes and genotypes. Ann Neurol 43: 485–93.

55. Kumada T, Ito M, Miyajima T, et al. (2005) Multi-institutional study on the correlation between chromosomal abnormalities and epilepsy. Brain Dev—NPN 27: 127–34.

56. Butler JV, Whittington JE, Holland AJ. (2002) Prevalence of, and risk factors for, physical ill-health in people with Prader-Willi syndrome: A population-based study. Dev Med Child Neurol 44: 248–55.

57. Shapira NA, Lessig MC, Murphy TK, et al. (2002) Topiramate attenuates self-injurious behavior in Prader-Willi Syndrome. Inter J Neuropsychopharmacol 5: 141–5.

58. Smathers SA, Wilson JG, Nigro MA, et al. (2003) Topiramate effectiveness in Prader-Willi syndrome. Pediatr Neurol 28: 130–3.

59. Shapira NA, Lessig MC, LewisMH, et al. (2004) Effects of topiramate in adults with Prader-Willi syndrome. Am J Ment Retard 109: 301–9

60. Battaglia A, Battaglia A. (2005) The inv dup(15) or idic(15) syndrome: A clinically recognisable neurogenetic disorder. Brain and Development. 27: 365–9.

61. Ahlsén G, Gillberg IC, Lindblom R. et al. (1994)Tuberous sclerosis in Western Sweden. A population study of cases with early childhood onset. Arch Neurology. 51: 76–81.

62. Hunt A. (1993) Development, behaviour and seizures in 300 cases of tuberous sclerosis. J Intellect Disabil Res 37: 41–51.

63. Gillberg C. (1995) Clinical child neuropsychiatry.Cambridge University Press. Cambridge, UK:

64. Riikonen R, Simell O. (1990) Tuberous sclerosis and infantile spasms. Dev Med Child Neurol 32: 203–9.

65. Guerreiro MM, Andermann F, Andermann E, et al. (1998) Surgical treatment of epilepsy in tuberous sclerosis: strategies and results in 18 patients. Neurology 51: 1263–9.

66. Stafstrom CE, Patxot OF, Gilmore HE, et al. (1991) Seizures in children with Down syndrome: Etiology, characteristics and outcome. Dev Med Child Neurol 33: 191–200.

67. Lazarowski A, Lubieniecki F, Camarero S, et al. (2006). New proteins configure a brain drug resistance map in tuberous sclerosis. Pediatr Neurol 34: 20–4.

68. Riikonen R, Donner M. (1979) Incidence and etiology of infantile spasms from 1960 to 1976: A population study in Finland.Dev Med Child Neurol 21: 333–43.

69. Guerrini R, Genton P, Bureau M, et al. (1990) Reflex seizures are frequent in patients with Down syndrome and epilepsy. Epilepsia 31: 406–17.

70. Brown SW. (2002) Epilepsy. In: Prasher VP, Janicki MP, (eds) Physical health of adults with intellectual disabilities. Blackwell Publishing; Oxford: 133–59.

71. Pueschel SM, Louis S. McKnight P. (1991) Seizure disorders in Down syndrome. Arch Neurol 84: 318–20.

72. Lai F, Williams RS.(1989) A prospective study of Alzheimer disease in Down syndrome. Arch Neurol 46: 849–53.

73. Evenhuis HM.(1990) The natural history of dementia in Down's syndrome. Arch Neurol 47: 263–7.

74. Genton P, Paglia G. (1994) É pilepsie myoclonique sénile (senile myoclonic epilepsy). Epilepsies 6: 5–11.
75. SabersA,(1999) Epilepsy in Down Syndrome. In: Sillanpaa M, Gram L, Johannessen SI, Tomsom T (eds). Epilepsy & mental retardation. Wrightson Biomedical Publishing, Petersfield, Hampshire, UK: 41–5.
76. Glauser TA, Morita DA. (2002) Lennox-Gastaut syndrome. In: Devinsky O, Westbrook LE (eds). Epilepsy and developmental disabilities. Butterworth-Heinemann, Woburn, MA: 65–78.
77. Trevathan E, Murphy CC, Yeargin-Allsopp M. (1997) Prevalence and descriptive epidemiology of Lennox-Gastaut syndrome among Atlanta children.Epilepsia 38: 1283–8.
78. Jenkins LK, Brown SW. (1990) The value of syndrome classification in childhood epilepsy. Acta Neurologica Scandinavica 82 (Suppl)133:–10.

Chapter 4
Diagnosis of Epilepsy in Persons with Intellectual Disabilities

P. Martin

Introduction

As has been highlighted in Chapter 3, epileptic seizures occur more frequently in persons with intellectual disabilities (ID) than in individuals from the general population.[1] This is especially true in severe and profound ID. The incidence of epilepsies may be even greater when ID is due to a specific syndrome like tuberous sclerosis complex (TSC). In some disorders and syndromes the probability of seizures is age dependent or linked to coexisting disorders — e.g. a very high likelihood of seizures in Angelman Syndrome during infancy and childhood, or as part of dementia in Alzheimer's disease seen in older persons with Down syndrome.[2–6]

This must be kept in mind when a patient with ID presents first with a questionable seizure. The possibility of the fit in question being truly epileptic in nature must not be estimated in relation to the whole population but to the cohort of persons with ID of the same severity or cause. In general the likelihood of a paroxysmal event in a person with an ID being an epileptic disorder is higher than in individuals from the general population. The incidence, however, of nonepileptic motor or behavior paroxysms is greater in the ID population.

The Patient's Medical History

The history of a patient with epilepsy and ID must cover information about

1. The onset and course of the epilepsy.
2. Seizure semiology, including subjective aspects of the seizures.
3. Affect and behavior during the prodromal and postictal periods.
4. Daytime distribution of the seizures.
5. Severity of the seizures and seizure hazards.
6. Specific seizure precipitating factors in the individual patient.
7. Anticonvulsive efficiency and tolerability of the medication (present and past).
8. Behavioral and psychiatric disorders of the patient and family members.

V.P. Prasher, M.P. Kerr (eds.) *Epilepsy and Intellectual Disabilities*,
DOI: 10.1007/978-1-84800-259-3_4, © Springer Science+Business Media, LLC 2008

In many cases it is very difficult to get sufficient information on the history of an adult patient with ID reaching back to infancy and childhood. Further, in persons with severe ID it is impossible to obtain an accurate history from the patient her- or himself. Often there are no informants who oversee the course of the seizure disorder over the whole lifespan of the individual with ID.

To classify not only the epileptic syndrome but also the cause of the ID in given patient it is often essential to get information on the early evolution of epileptic seizures. This applies, for example, to patients with severe myoclonic epilepsy in infancy (Dravet's syndrome), where initially prolonged, generalized, or unilateral clonic seizures are typically triggered by fever occurring in normal infants.[7] Psychomotor delay becomes progressively evident from the second year on and correlates with an initial high frequency of convulsive seizures. Another example would be an epileptic syndrome caused by hypothalamic hamartomas associated with cognitive deterioration, behavioral problems, and precocious puberty in many cases. Gelastic seizures occur in almost all children with hypothalamic hamartoma but are not a prominent feature of epilepsy in adult patients.[8,9] Therefore, gelastic seizures in the history would give an important hint about a hypothalamic hamartoma being the cause of ID in a patient with epilepsy and behavior problems.

It may seem impossible to obtain information on the subjective experience of seizures from a person with severe ID. A competent physician should be able to allow for this when he or she intends to identify details of the seizures in the severely impaired person. There can be short verbalizations ("ah," "fear," "oh no," etc.) and, in some patients, behavioral changes (clinging to an attendant person, fearful face, etc.) that constantly appear at the beginning of a seizure, followed by impairment of consciousness and motor symptoms. In either event those symptoms are an indication of auras or simple partial seizures. Their presence leads to the presumption that the patient suffers from localization-related epilepsy, and may be crucial considerations when epilepsy surgery is considered. The existence and duration of auras are also important with regard to the patient's ability to protect her- or himself in the initial state of a seizure where self-harm may result (e.g., drop seizure). Sometimes, if the symptoms of an aura last long enough, it may enable the caregivers to administer emergency medication before the simple partial seizure progresses to, for example, a tonic clonic seizure. In some instances, when auras consist of a feeling of fear, an anxiety disorder may develop in a patient.[10] In those cases, carefully working up of the seizure semiology gives the crucial information for interpreting a coexisting psychiatric disease.

Many patients with epilepsy eventually experience prodromal changes of their mood and behavior that signal the impending seizure to their caregivers. Symptoms frequently seen are aggression, dysphoria, or hyperactivity. Elation, increased speech production, and strengthened attentiveness also occur, as well as other emotional and behavioral changes. Different affective states, often amelioration of the mood and affability, can be seen in the postictal period. Prodromal and postictal symptoms, as opposed to the epileptic aura, are not part of the electroclinical seizure and are not accompanied by ictal neurophysiological changes. The subjective facet of the epileptic disorder is important to help understand any prodromal or postictal affective changes. In most of the patients with an ID this would only be possible to assess during the caregiver interview.[11–13]

Information on seizure semiology should enable the physician to differentiate between epileptic and psychogenic nonepileptic seizures (PNES). Table 4.1 lists semiologic details that can help to distinguish PNES from epileptic seizures. In patients with ID it is likewise of importance to make out other paroxysmal nonepileptic motor and behavior events (Table 4.2). Although this information has already been mentioned in Chapter 1 it will be discussed in more detail in this chapter.

Information about night-time distribution of seizures is especially difficult in those patients who live in settings which do not provide observation during the night. Sleep- and awakening-related seizures are missed by the caregivers in those cases. It is, however, important to know about seizures during sleep and waking up. In many cases there maybe less complicating hazards because the patient cannot

Table 4.1 Clinical characteristics of psychogenic nonepileptic seizures (PNES)

Symptoms in PNES

Long duration (frequently more than 10 minutes)
Status of psychogenic nonepileptic seizures (PNES) are frequent
Predominantly motor behavior
- Diminished rhythmicity
- Beating and kicking movements
- Pelvic thrusting
- Head reclination
- Discontinuous; crescendo-decrescendo pattern
- Missing anatomical logics
- Less uniform (different seizures of the same patient)

Eyes closed/screwed up
Pupillary reaction to light
Reaction to sensory stimuli during the seizure
No or little postictal exhaustion
Enuresis and encopresis may happen
Nearly never lateral tongue bites

Table 4.2 Paroxysmal nonepileptic motor and behavior events that can be confused with epileptic fits

Neurological/Cardiovascular	Psychiatric/Behavioral
Exaggerated startle response	Tics
Sleep disorders/parasomnias	Aggression
Syncopes	Stereotype movements
Falls (other causes like disorders of gait and balance)	Paranoid and hallucinatory experiences leading to "absorbed" absence-like behavior
Dsykinetic movements	Anxiety behavior
	Behavioral expression of pain and other somatic complaints
	Elation and laughter

fall and hurt her- or himself while resting in bed. Sleep-related seizures, however, compromise the sleep effectiveness and quality, thus leading to daytime sleepiness, as well as to behavioral and cognitive changes when the patient is awake.[14,15] The physician should know about the habitual sleep position of a patient experiencing seizures during sleep as well as about the size and material of her or his pillow. This may aid the risk assessment of asphyxiation during a sleep-related seizure.

Other important questions concerning hazards of sleep related seizures would be: Is there an initial cry that warns caregivers when a seizure takes place, and does the patient move significantly while having a seizure so as to make an epilepsy alarm system suggestive, or is she or he in danger of falling out of bed while having a seizure?

The severity of seizures experienced by a patient can be assessed, in addition to other criteria, by the duration of the dimming or loss of consciousness, absence of protective warning time, and the danger of falling. Seizures with falls are tonic, atonic, tonic-clonic, or, more rarely, myoclonic. Tonic seizures are very frequently seen in epilepsy patients with a ID and often precede a psychomotor evolution of the seizure in this patient group. Of seizures with falls, atonic seizures lead most frequently to severe injuries.[16] Almost half of the patients who experience epileptic drop attacks have ID.[17]

As part of the assessment of seizures, it is important to assess for precipitating factors. Not only in infancy and childhood but also in adolescence and adulthood seizures may be precipitated by infectious diseases and fever.[18] In some patients this can be a regular and frequent occurrence. The excerbation of epilepsy by fever is characteristic of individual syndromes like Angelman syndrome or Dravet's syndrome.[7,19] The contrary condition can also be true — improvement in the seizure disorder during febrile infections.[20]

There are numerous other seizure-inducing factors, such as many different sensory stimuli, e.g., flashing lights, other visual and acoustic stimuli, or putting one's hands into warm water or touching particular kinds of fabrics. The physician has to know about specific seizure-precipitating factors in his or her epilepsy patients and whether or not there are hints of a possible self-induction of seizures.[21–23] Other important factors leading to an augmentation of seizure frequency are discomfort and stress or conflicts at the residential home or working place.[18] A worsening of the epilepsy may also be due to sleep disturbances of any kind, and seizures and antiepileptic treatment are associated with sleep disruption.[24] Neither stress nor the sleep disturbances are often reported spontaneously by the patient or their caregivers; therefore, the physician has to actively inquire about those factors.

The potential adverse effects of antiepileptic medication on a person with ID should de considered prior to initiating the medication. Almost every antiepileptic drug has potential adverse effects on emotional states and behavior. Some substances, such as barbiturates, topiramate, or vigabatrin, are particularly prone to exert undesired psychiatric effects. When starting with a new drug, the risk of newly developing or enhanced emotional or behavioral disorders in an individual patient can be estimated by taking account of several risk factors: difficult-to-treat epilepsy, anticonvulsive polypharmacy, rapid titration, and high dosages, as well as an individual and family history of previous psychiatric disorders.[25] The latter have to be assessed carefully before starting with a new substance.

Diagnostic Evaluation: Aims and Questions to be Answered

Together with historical data, the diagnostic evaluation must answer several questions. First, it must determine whether a paroxysmal event is of epileptic nature and whether the patient should be diagnosed with epilepsy. Second, if the diagnosis is epilepsy, it must be assigned to an epilepsy syndrome (see Table 4.3). Third, a possible structural cause of the seizures (and ID) should be looked for, as well as a possible underlying genetic disorder (with epilepsy and ID).

Classification with a particular epileptic syndrome provides contingent prognostic and therapeutic implications. Structural lesions of the brain indicate not only a possible epileptogenic lesion but also give information on the causes of disorders (e.g., motor, visual, etc.) associated with the ID and epilepsy. The diagnosis of a syndrome, a genetically determined developmental disorder of the brain, or a neurocutaneous syndrome form the basis of genetic counseling of the family (see Tables 4.4 and 4.5).

As part of the ongoing assessment of epilepsy, other associated disorders should be identified by the clinical examination. These can affect the occurrence and the course of epilepsies in persons with ID (see Chapter 3). For example, epilepsy is one of the most common disorders associated with cerebral palsy (CP). Population-based studies and clinical series revealed a ratio of 30–40% of concomitant epilepsy in children with CP. Epilepsy is significantly more common in patients with severe CP and with ID.[42] Epilepsy in hemiplegic CP can be difficult to treat in many cases.[43] In autistic persons the chance of experiencing an unprovoked seizure is substantially higher than in the general population (up to 39% in autism). There is an elevation in risk in early childhood and another subsequent increase in adolescence in autistic persons, i.e., a bimodal age distribution of epilepsy incidence.[44,45]

In rarer cases, inborn metabolic diseases have to be considered in the etiological diagnosis of ID and epilepsy, but they will not be discussed in this chapter.

Table 4.3 Epilepsy Syndromes associated with ID.[26]

Epileptic syndrome	
Early infantile epileptic encephalopathy with suppression-burst	Ohtahara's syndrome
Early (neonatal) myoclonic encephalopathy	
Infantile spasms	West syndrome
	Lennox-Gastaut syndrome
Severe myoclonic epilepsy in infancy	Dravet's syndrome
Epilepsy with myoclonic absences	
Epilepsy with myoclonic-astatic seizures	Doose's syndrome

Table 4.4 Cerebral developmental disorders and their presently known genetic causes[27-30]

Disorder	Gene (localization)
Lissencephaly type I, Subcortical band heterotopia	LIS 1 (17p13.3), DCX (X q22.3-q23)
X chromosomal lissencephaly with abnormal genitalia (XLAG)	ARX (Xp22.12)
Lissencephaly with cerebellar hypoplasia	RELN (7q22), VLDLR (9q24)
Cobblestone lissencephaly (in, e.g., Walker Warburg disease, Muscle eye brain disease, Fukuyama disease)	POMT1 (9q34.1), POMT2 (14q24.3), POMTGnT1 (1p33-p34), FKRP (19q13.3), FCMD (9q31), LARGE (22q12.3)
Holoprosencephaly	SIX3 (2p21), SHH (7q36), TGIF (18pter-q11), ZIC2 (13q32), ZIC1-ZIC4? (3p24-pter), forkhead homologue (13q12-14), thyroid transcription factor-1? (14q13), homologue to mouse coloboma (20q13), ? (1q42-qter), ? (5p), ? (6q26-qter), PTCH (9q22.3), DHCR (11q13); trisomy 13, trisomy 18
Microcephaly	MCPH1 (8p23), CDK5RAP2 (9q34), ASPM (1q31), CENPJ (13q12.2)
Periventricular nodular heterotopia	FLNA (Xq28)
Autosomal recessive periventricular heterotopia with microcephaly	ARFGEF2 (20q13.12)
Polymicrogyria (bilateral frontoparietal)	GPR56 (16q13)

Table 4.5 Neurocutaneous syndromes associated with ID and epilepsy/seizures[31-41]

Syndrome	Prevalence	Incidence of ID	Incidence of Epilepsy/Seizures
Tuberous sclerosis complex	1 : 30 000	38–53%	78%
Neurofibromatosis I	1 : 3000	30–45%	3-12%
Sturge-Weber syndrome	1 : 10 000	70–75%	80%
Linear nevus sebaceus syndrome	500 cases described	61%	67%
Hypomelanosis Ito	Unclear 1: 3000 children in a pediatric service	57–70%	37-53%
Incontinentia pigmenti	1 : 40 000	7 %	9%
Proteus syndrome	< 1 : 10^6	Described	Described
Neurocutaneous melanosis	$1 : 2 \cdot 10^5 - 5 \cdot 10^5$	Described	Described
Basal cell nevus syndrome	1 : 57 000	Described	Described
Chediak-Higashi syndrome	200 cases described	Described	Described

Electroencephalography (EEG)

Besides a detailed and comprehensive history, an EEG assessment is the most important diagnostic method in the diagnosis of epilepsy. Obtaining an EEG recording in patients with ID is difficult and time consuming in many cases. This is true especially in timid and restless persons. In those cases it is often helpful to customize the patient slowly to the situation. Providing a familiar situation by allowing the patient to hear her or his favorite music or to bring a familiar object would have a calming influence.

It is advisable to keep the time the EEG assistant takes to apply the electrodes to the head as brief as possible. Among the many different EEG electrode application techniques, electrocaps are especially suited for patients with ID and/or behavioral problems. They are made of an elastic fabric with electrodes firmly integrated into the caps. Electrocaps are available in different seizes and provide a significantly shorter application time than other systems. Their main drawback is that their fixed electrodes can be placed only roughly adjusted to the individual head size and shape according to the international 10–20 positioning system. Many patients with ID will not cooperate sufficiently so as to obtain effects of hyperventilation on the EEG. Using a wind wheel is a practicable tool in those cases.

When an EEG is performed to evaluate patients with suspected seizures the first recording should be performed for at least 20 minutes and should, when possible, involve hyperventilation and intermittent photic stimulation.[46] There continues to be debate on the degree of usefulness of the EEG in the diagnosis of epilepsy in persons with ID[47]; however, clinicians in their day-to-day practice still prefer to undertake an EEG assessment.

As it is very unlikely to record a patient's habitual seizure during routine EEG, interictal epileptiform discharges (IEDs) are the most significant EEG changes when epilepsy is in question. Interictal epileptiform discharges are rare in individuals, especially adult persons, without epilepsy. In patients without epilepsy (in the community) they are found in 3.3% with no provoked or unprovoked seizures during follow-up.[47] The occurrence of IEDs in selected populations of healthy adults is reported to be much lower.[48]

A first EEG recorded from patients with epilepsy shows IEDs in only 20–50%.[47,48] The yield of EEG can be substantially increased by repeating recordings and activation techniques like hyperventilation, intermittent photic stimulation, and sleep deprivation.[49] Hyperventilation is more effective in generalized epilepsies, where it provokes 3/s spike wave activity; hyperventilation seems also able to enhance slow spike and wave activity in symptomatic generalized epilepsies, which occur frequently in persons with ID.[50] Intermittent photic stimulation can elicit different EEG responses, of which the photoparoxysmal response (generalized paroxysms with spike-/polyspike and slow waves) is specifically associated with epilepsy. It is most probably a genetic trait and is particularly seen in young patients with generalized epilepsies.[49] Sleep EEG increases the sensitivity of EEG by a substantial amount of 30–70% (including a sampling effect, due to the additional sleep EEG with a longer recording time), sometimes even up to 90% when it is recorded after sleep deprivation.[49,51]

Among EEG changes in patients with ID and epilepsy there are various typical patterns characterizing (1) a specific epileptic syndrome, (2) a peculiar disorder of the cortical development, or (3) genetic syndromes associated with ID and epilepsy. Hypsarrhythmia is the specific EEG correlate of infantile spasms (West syndrome).

Slow spike and wave activity is usual in the Lennox Gastaut syndrome but is of little specificity, whereas sleep-related frontal spike bursts (runs of rapid spikes) with and without tonic seizures are much more distinctive.[52,53] Ohtahara's syndrome shows characteristic EEG features with suppression-burst pattern, where bursts last 2–6s and comprise high-voltage slow waves intermingled with spikes.[54] Dravet's syndrome, myoclonic astatic epilepsy, or the syndrome of myoclonic absences do not show any characteristic interictal EEG pattern; EEG photosensitivity, however, is very frequently seen in children with Dravet's disease.[7,55,56]

Several distinct structural lesions of the brain that cause epilepsy (and ID) show characteristic changes of the interictal EEG. In Sturge-Weber syndrome the most consistent interictal EEG finding is a depression of amplitude over the affected hemisphere or parts of the hemisphere. Epileptiform activity appears frequently over the contralateral hemisphere or, in children, as a bilateral synchronous paroxysmal activity.[57] Interictal EEG patterns in focal cortical dysplasia consist of continuous or quasicontinuous rhythmic spiking or repetitive spiking in many patients.[58,59]

In hemimegalencephaly, background activity is often asymmetric with pathological alpha activation (higher amplitudes over the hemimegalencephalic hemisphere) and loss of physiological activity (e.g., sleep spindles) on the side of the pathology as well as suppression burst activity and/or hemihypsarrhythmia.[60,61] There are rather uniform EEG findings in bilateral subcortical band heterotopia (double cortex syndrome): more or less slow background activity and paroxysmal high-voltage bilateral synchronous slow activity with intermingled spikes and sharp waves as well as sporadic focal epileptiform activity.[62] The EEG in Type I lissencephaly frequently shows an absence of the normal distribution of local activities; diffuse, rhythmic fast alpha and beta activity; high-voltage focal, multifocal, or bisynchronous spike wave activity.[63]

There are several genetic syndromes associated with ID and epilepsy in which frequently appearing and typical EEG patterns are described. In Angelman syndrome (AS) characteristic EEG patterns do not differentiate between patients with and without seizures. The most frequent finding, independent of the patient's age, is high-amplitude 2–3 Hz rhythmic activity over the frontal regions with interspersed epileptiform elements. In childhood high-amplitude rhythmic 4–6 Hz activity over the occipital regions with associated spikes, facilitated by eye closure, is a frequent pattern in AS.[64]

In Wolf-Hirschhorn syndrome paroxysms of bisynchronous 2–3Hz waves of high amplitude associated with sharp waves and spikes of lower amplitude seem to be a characteristic EEG pattern, enhanced during drowsiness and sleep.[65,66] In Kabuki syndrome, a clinical entity in which a consistent genetic abnormality has not been defined yet, characteristic EEG findings with temporo-occipital spikes (during sleep) are described.[67] In many other syndromes associated with ID and epilepsy no characteristic EEG patterns could be found.

Long-term EEG or video-EEG monitoring can add substantial information and serve as the gold standard in relation to many clinical questions:

1. To differentiate between epileptic seizures and nonepileptic paroxysmal events.
2. To reveal sleep-related seizures.
3. To obtain more information on the semiology of seizures.
4. To obtain information on the electroclinical correlation of seizures with respect to epilepsy surgery.
5. To relate (subtle) seizures to possible cognitive impairment.

All aspects mentioned above can be applied to patients with ID. In individuals with severe ID, especially in Rett's syndrome, paroxysmal (repetitive, hyperactive) behavior is frequently mistaken for epileptic events. In many cases a correct diagnosis is only achieved by video-EEG monitoring, where, on the other hand, subtle seizures not previously recognized by the caregivers can be uncovered.[68] Even in cases with multifocal cerebral lesions and multifocal interictal epileptiform discharges, TSC ictal recordings together with magnetic resonance imaging (MRI) can identify the focus of seizure activity. Epilepsy surgery is beneficial in many patients with TSC who become seizure free after resection of the epileptogenic tuber.[69]

Neuroimaging

Magnetic resonance imaging serves as the method of first choice, not only to identify a possible epileptogenic lesion but also to reveal the causes of ID and other associated disorders (Figures 4.1 and 4.2).

The advantages of MRI over computed tomography (CT) are numerous. First of all, the sensitivity and specificity of CT in patients with epilepsy to detect and characterize anomalies and possible epileptogenic lesions is far too low; in addition, CT uses ionizing radiation. Computed tomography, however, has a higher scan speed and therefore is still crucial in emergency situations. Neuroimaging goals are

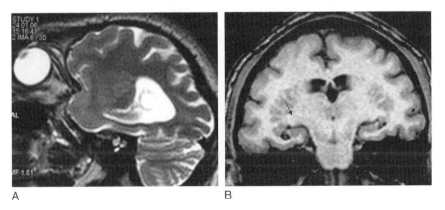

A   B

Fig. 4.1 MR images of a patient with extreme microcephaly, learning disability, and epilepsy. (A) Sagittal T2-weighted inage (compare the size of the eye with the brain size!). (B) T1-weighted image showing conglomerate masses of gray matter (heterotopias) between ventricular walls/basal ganglia and the cortex *(arrows)*

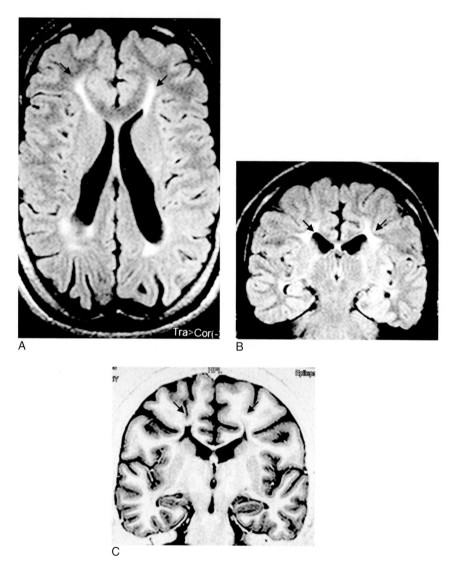

Fig. 4.2 MR images of a patient with a history of preterm birth and learning disability, cerebral palsy and epilepsy, showing bilateral periventricular leukomalacia *(arrows)*. (A) Axial fluid attenuated inversion recovery (FLAIR) images showing periventricular white matter abnormalities around the frontal horns and the trigone of both sides. (B) Coronal FLAIR sequence and (C) Coronal T1-weighted inversion recovery sequence, both showing residual core cavities of periventricular hypoxic-ischemic lesions

to identify underlying lesions and to help in the formulation of syndromic and etiological causes of epilepsy and associated disorders (ID, CP, etc.) in a given patient. To detect a circumscribed lesion in an epilepsy patient with refractory epilepsy implicates the possibility of surgical treatment (Figures 4.3 to 4.5) .

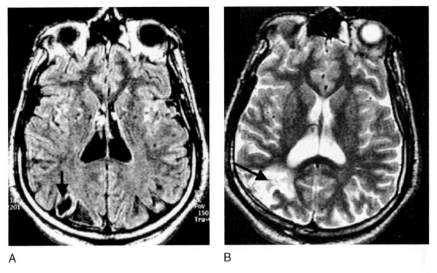

A   B

Fig. 4.3 MR images of a right parietal dysembryoblastic neuroepithelial tumor *(arrow)* identified as an epileptogenic lesion. (A) FLAIR sequence before and (B) T2-weighted sequence after surgical resection *(arrow)*

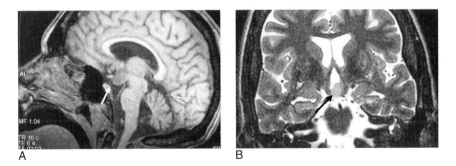

A   B

Fig. 4.4 MR images showing a hypothalamic hamartoma *(arrow)* in a patient with learning disability, drug-resistant epilepsy, and severe aggressive behavioral disturbances as well as precocious puberty. The patient underwent gamma knife radiosurgery resulting in substantially better seizure control and improvement of behavior. (A) T1-weighted sagittal and (B) coronal T2-weighted images

Defined disorders of cerebral development like lissencephaly and band heterotopias, polymicrogyria, and hemimegalencephaly or cerebral lesions in neurocutaneous syndromes are demonstrated by MRI and can be frequently traced back to peculiar genetic factors (Figures 4.6 to 4.8; see also Table 4.4).

MRI protocols in patients with epilepsy should include T1-weighted and T2-weighted sequences as well as FLAIR (fluid-attenuated inversion recovery)

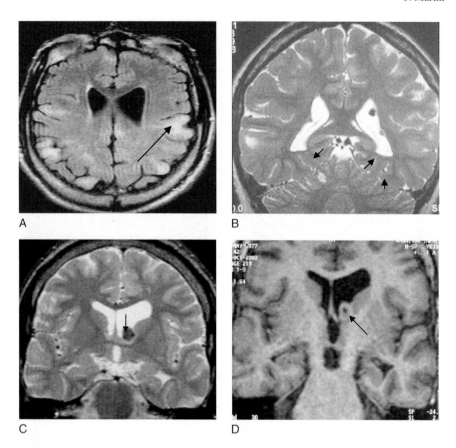

Fig. 4.5 MRI scans of a patient with tuberous sclerosis complex. (A) Axial fluid attenuated inversion recovery images (FLAIR) showing multiple cortical tubers *(arrow)*. (B) Coronal T2-weighted image demonstrating multiple subependymal nodules *(arrows)* of the trigona. (C, D) Coronal T2-weighted and T1-weighted images of a subependymal giant cell astrocytoma at the level of the foramen of Monro *(arrow)*

sequences, and T1-weighted inversion recovery sequences in two or three orthogonal planes (axial, coronal, and sagittal) with a slice thickness of 1.5 to 3.0 mm. The sequences should include volume acquisition with thin partition size (< 1.5-2.0mm) to allow reformatting and three-dimensional reconstruction. Gradient echo sequences with high sensitivity to differences in magnetic susceptibility are suited to detect hemosiderin-containing and calcified lesions (e.g., in Sturge-Weber syndrome).[70],[71] In most cases patients are not able to keep still during the MRI examination. Therefore brief anesthesia will be necessary. This would be a convenient opportunity to perform other examinations such as lumbar puncture or ophthalmoscopy.

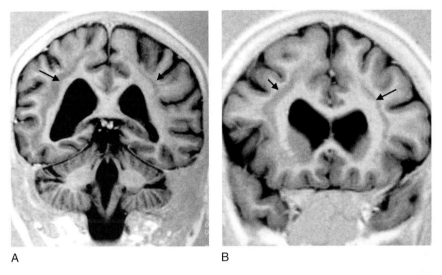

Fig. 4.6 Coronal T1-weighted inversion recovery sequences showing bands of ectopic neuronal tissue in the white matter of the cerebral hemispheres – band heterotopias – which are broader on the right in this patient. (A) Parietal section and (B) frontal section

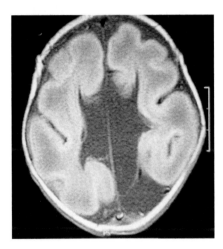

Fig. 4.7 Axial T1-weighted MR image of a 9-month-old male patient with severe developmental disability, catastrophic epilepsy, micropenis, and hypospadiasis, diagnosed with X-linked lissencephaly with abnormal genitalia (XLAG) and with a mutation of the Aristaless-related homeobox gene (ARX). The image shows typical and severe pachygyria, more in the posterior than in the frontal cortical regions, with moderately thickened cortex and complete agenesis of the corpus callosum

Other neuroimaging techniques, such as single-photon emission CT (SPECT), positron emission tomography (PET), magnetic resonance spectroscopy (MRS), functional MRI (fMRI), and magnetoencephalography (MEG), are additional tools in the context of preoperative workup but are beyond the scope of this chapter.

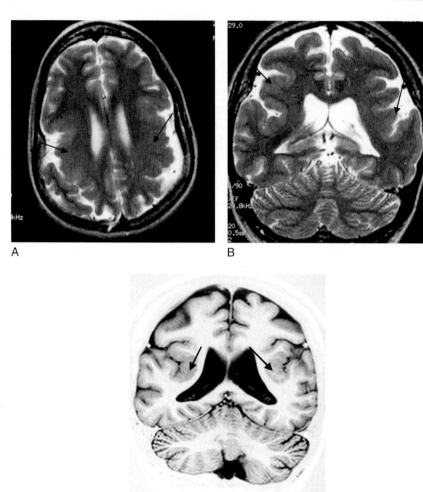

Fig. 4.8 MRI morphology of perisylvian polymicrogyria. (A) Axial and (B) coronal T2-weighted images showing widespread bilateral frontoparietal polymicrogyrias surrounding the Sylvian fissure *(arrows)*. (C) Smaller circumscribed polymicrogyrias in the depth of the lateral sulcus on both sides *(arrows)*

Summary/Conclusion

The history, clinical examination, EEG, and MRI are the most important elements in patients with ID and epilepsy. Though the prevalence of epilepsies is substantially higher in individuals with ID than in the general population, it may be more difficult to differentiate nonepileptic paroxysmal motor and behavioral events from epileptic seizures. The diagnostic process, in particular, must cover the issues of possible hazards of fits, precipitating factors, and also possible subjective aspects of seizures. Seizure semiology, EEG findings, and structural changes on MRI scans may help to judge whether an individual patient suffers from surgical remediable epilepsy.

In many patients, particularly in those who live in residential homes, seizures, especially sleep-related fits, are missed but can be detected during long time EEG-video monitoring. All diagnostic steps are in most cases more difficult to perform and more time consuming than in patients without ID and require a special training of physicians and other health professionals.

More frequently than in persons without ID, the diagnostic process, including a thorough clinical examination, must aim at an etiological and syndromal (genetic) classification, thus providing a basis of further prognostic statements, therapeutic decisions, and family genetic counseling.

References

1. Morgan CL, Baxter H, Kerr MP. (2003) Prevalence of epilepsy and associated health service utilization and mortality among patients with intellectual disability. Am J Ment Retard 108: 293–300.
2. Lhatoo SD, Sander JWAS. (2001) The epidemiology of epilepsy and learning disability. Epilepsia 42 (Suppl. 1):6–9.
3. Matson JL, Bamburg JW, Mayville EA, et al. (1999) Seizure disorders in people with intellectual disability: An analysis of differences in social functioning, adaptive functioning and maladaptive behaviours. J Intellect Disabil Res 43: 531–9.
4. Gómez MR. (1999) Natural history of cerebral tuberous sclerosis. In: Gómez MR, Sampson JR, Whittemore VH (eds.). Tuberous sclerosis complex. New York, Oxford: Oxford University Press, 1999, 29–46.
5. Mendez M. (2005) Down syndrome, Alzheimer's disease and seizures. Brain Dev 27: 246–52.
6. Valente KD, Koiffmann CP, Fridman C, et al. (2006) Epilepsy in patients with Angelman syndrome caused by deletion of the chromosome 15q11–13. Arch Neurol 63: 122–8.
7. Dravet C, Bureau M, Oguni H, et al. (2002) Severe myoclonic epilepsy in infancy (Dravet syndrome). In: Roger J, Breau M, Dravet C et al., (eds.). Epileptic syndromes in infancy child-hood and Adolescence. Eastleigh, UK: John Libbey, 81–103.
8. Mullatti N, Selway R, Nashef L, et al. (2003) The clinical spectrum of epilepsy in children and adults with hypothalamic hamartoma. Epilepsia 44: 1310–19.
9. Berkovic SF, Kuzniecky RI, Andermann F. (1997) Human epileptogenesis and hypothalamic hamartomas: New lessons from an experiment of nature. Epilepsia 38: 1–3.
10. Kohler CG, Carran MA, Bilker W, et al. (2001) Association of fear auras with mood and anxiety disorders after temporal lobectomy. Epilepsia 42: 674–81.
11. Kanner AM, Kuzniecky R. (2001) Psychiatric phenomena as an expression of postictal and paraictal events. In: Ettinger AB, Kanner AM (eds). Psychiatric issues in epilepsy: A practical guide to diagnosis and treatment. Philadelphia: Lippincott Williams&Wilkins, 163–79.
12. Schachter SC. (2001) Aggressive behaviour in epilepsy. In: Ettinger AB, Kanner AM (eds). Psychiatric issues in epilepsy: A practical guide to diagnosis and treatment. Philadelphia: Lippincott Williams & Wilkins, 201–14.
13. Blanchet P, Frommer GP. (1986) Mood change preceding epileptic seizures. J Nerv Ment Dis 174: 471–6.

14. Brylewski J, Wiggs L (1999) Sleep problems and daytime challenging behaviour in a community-based sample of adults with intellectual disability. J Intellect Disabil Res 43: 504–12.
15. Lindblom N, Heiskala H, Kaski M, et al. (2001) Neurological impairments and sleep-wake bahaviour among mentally retarded. J Sleep Res 10: 309–18.
16. Nakken KO, Lossius R. (1993) Seizure-related injuries in multihandicapped patients with therapy-resistant epilepsy. Epilepsia 34: 836–40.
17. Tinuper P, Cerullo A, Marini C, et al. (1998) Epileptic drop attacks in partial epilepsy: Clinical features, evolution, and prognosis. J Neurol Neurosurg Psychiatry 64: 231–7.
18. Frucht MM, Quigg M, Schwaner C, et al. (2000) Distribution of seizure precipitants among epilepsy syndromes. Epilepsia 200: 41(12): 1534–39.
19. Galvan-Manso M, Campistol J, Conill J et al. (2005) Analysis of the characteristics of epilepsy in 37 patients with the molecular diagnosis of Angelman syndrome. Epileptic Disord 7: 19–25.
20. Ernst JP. (2004) Fever can suppress epilepsy seizures. Epilepsia 45(Suppl.3): 199.
21. Bebek N, Baykan B, Gurses C, et al. (2006) Self-induction behavior in patients with photosensitive and hot water epilepsy: A comparative study from a tertiary epilepsy center in Turkey. Epilepsy Behav 9: 317–26.
22. Ng BY. (2002) Psychiatric aspects of self-induced epileptic seizures. Aust NZJ Psychiatry 36: 534–43.
23. Binnie CD. (1988) Self-induction of seizures: The ultimate non-compliance. Epilepsy Res (Suppl) 1: 153–8.
24. Bazil CW. (2003) Epilepsy and sleep disturbance. Epilepsy Behav 4(Suppl. 2): S39–45.
25. Schmitz B. (1999) Psychiatric syndromes related to antiepileptic drugs. Epilepsia 40(Suppl. 10): S65–70.
26. Engel J. (2006) ILAE classification of epilepsy syndromes. Epilepsy Res 70(Suppl. 1): S5–10.
27. Uyanik G, Hehr U, Martin P, et al. (2005) Genetics of cerebral malformations: Neuronal migration disorders. Med M Geist M Behind 2: 9–21.
28. Cohen MM. (2006) Holoprosencephaly: Clinical, anatomic,and molecular dimensions. 76: 658–73.
29. Ten Donkelaar HJ, Lammens M, Cruysberg JRM, et al. (2006) Development and developmental disorders of the forebrain. In: Ten Donkelaar HJ, Lammens M, Hori A (eds). Clinical neuro-embryology. Berlin, Heidelberg, New York: Springer, 345–411.
30. Barkovich AJ, Kuzniecky RI, Jackson GD, et al. (2005) A developmental and genetic classification for malformations of cortical development. Neurology 65: 1873–87.
31. Warkany J, Lemire RJ, Cohen MM. (1981) Mental retardation and congenital malformations of the central nervous system. Chicago, London: Year Book Medical Publishers.
32. Friedman JM. (2002) Neurofibromatosis 1: Clinical manifestations and diagnostic criteria. J Child Neurol 17: 548–54.
33. Shepherd CW. (1999) The epidemiology of the tuberous sclerosis complex. In: Gómez MR, Sampson JR, Whittemore VH (eds). Tuberous sclerosis complex. New York, Oxford: Oxford University Press, 24–8.
34. Cross JH. (2005) Neurocutaneous syndromes and epilepsy — issues in diagnosis and management. Epilepsia 46(Suppl. 10): 17–23.
35. Barkovich AJ. (2000) Pediatric neuroimaging. 3rd ed. Philadelphia: Lippincott Williams & Wilkins.
36. Cohen MM. (2005) Proteus syndrome: An update. Am J Med Genet C Semin Med Genet 137: 38–52.
37. De Freitas GR, De Oliveira CP, Reis RS, et al. (1999) Seizures in Chediak-Higashi syndrome. Case report. Arq Neuropsiquiatr. 57(2B): 495–7.
38. Murphy MJ, Tenser RB. (1982) Nevoid basal cell carcinoma syndrome and epilepsy. Ann Neurol 11: 372–6.
39. Incontinentia pigmenti international foundation; http://imgen.bcm.tmc.edu/IPIF

40. Baker RS, Ross PA, Baumann RJ. (1987) Neurologic complications of epidermal nevus syndrome. Arch Neurol 44: 227–32.
41. Vujevich JJ, Mancini AJ. (2004) The epidermal nevus syndromes: Multisystem disorders. J Am Acad Dermatol 50: 957–61.
42. D`Amelio M, Shinnar S, Hauser WA. (2002) Epilepsy in children with mental retardation and cerebral palsy. In: Devinsky O, Westbrook LE (eds).Epilepsy and developmental disabilities. Boston, Oxford, Auckland: Butterworth Heinemann, 3–15.
43. Uvebrant P. (1988) Hemiplegic cerebral palsy, aetiology and outcome. Acta Paediatr Scand (Suppl): 345.
44. Tuchman RF, Rapin I. (2002) Epilepsy in autism. Lancet Neurol. 1: 352–8.
45. Danielsson S, Gillberg C, Billstedt E, et al. (2005) Epilepsy in young adults with autism: A prospective population-based follow-up study of 120 individuals diagnosed in childhood. Epilepsia 46: 918–23.
46. American Electroencephalographic Society Guidelines in EEG, 1–7 (revised 1985) (1986) J Clin Neurophysiol 3: 131–68.
47. Sam MC, So EL. (2001) Significance of epileptiform discharges in patients without epilepsy in the community. Epilepsia 42: 1273–8.
48. Verma A, Radtke R. (2006) EEG of partial seizures. J Clin Neurophysiol 23: 333–9.
49. Mendez OE, Brenner RP. (2006) Increasing the yield of EEG. J Clin Neurophysiol 23: 282–93.
50. Blume WT, David RB, Gómez MR. (1973) Generalized sharp and slow wave complexes. Associated clinical features and long-term follow-up. Brain 96: 353–63.
51. Leach JP, Stephen LJ, Salveta C, et al. (2006) Which electroencephalography (EEG) for epilepsy? The relative usefulness of different EEG protocols in patients with possible epilepsy. J Neurol Neurosurg Psychiatry 77: 1040–2.
52. Hirt HR. (1996) Nosology of Lennox-Gastaut Syndrome. Nervenarzt. 67: 109–22.
53. Beaumanoir A. (1981) Les limites nosologiques du syndrome de Lennox-Gastaut. Revue EEG Neurophysiol 11(3–4): 468–73.
54. Aicardi J, Ohtahara S. (2002) Severe neonatal epilepsies with suppression-burst pattern. In: Roger J, Breau M, Dravet C, et al. (eds). Epileptic syndromes in infancy childhood and adolescence. Eastleigh, UK: John Libbey, 33–44.
55. Guerrini R, Parmeggiani L, Kaminska A, et al. (2002) Myoclonic astatic epilepsy. In: Roger J, Breau M, Dravet C, et al. (eds). Epileptic syndromes in infancy, childhood and adolescence. Eastleigh, UK: John Libbey, 105–12.
56. Bureau M, Tassinari CA. (2002) The syndrome of myoclonic absences. In: Roger J, Breau M, Dravet C, et al. (eds). Epileptic syndromes in infancy, childhood and adolescence. Eastleigh, UK: John Libbey, 305–12.
57. Arzimanoglou A. (1997) The surgical treatment of Sturge-Weber syndrome with respect to its clinical spectrum. In: Tuxhorn I, Holthausen H, Boenik H (eds). Paediatric epilepsy syndromes and their surgical treatment. London: John Libbey, 353–63.
58. Palmini A, Gambardella A, Andermann F, et al. (1995) Intrinsic epileptogenicity of human dysplastic cortex as suggested by corticography and surgical results. Ann Neurol 37: 476–87.
59. Fauser S, Schulze-Bonhage A. (2006) Epileptogenicity of cortical dysplasia in temporal lobe dual pathology: An electrophysiological study with invasive recordings. Brain 129: 82–95.
60. Vigevano F, Fusco L, Holthausen H, et al. (1997) The morphological spectrum and variable clinical picture in children with hemimegalencephaly. In: Tuxhorn I, Holthausen H, Boenigk H (eds). Paediatric epilepsy syndromes and their surgical treatment. London: John Libbey, 377–91.
61. Di Rocco C, Battaglia D, Pietrini D, et al. (2006) Childs Nerv Syst 22: 852–66.
62. Martin P, Spreer J, Uyanik G, et al. (2002) Band heterotopia: Clinic, EEG, functional MRI (fMRI) and genetics. In: Korinthenberg R (ed). Aktuelle Neuropaediatrie. Nuernberg: Novartis Verlag, 469–76.

63. Sarnat HB. (1992) Cerebral dysgenesis, embryology and clinical expression. New York, Oxford: Oxford University Press.
64. Laan LA, Vein AA. (2005) Angelman syndrome: Is there a characteristic EEG? Brain Dev 27: 80–7.
65. Valente KD, Freitas A, Fiore LA, et al. (2003) A study of EEG and epilepsy profile in Wolf-Hirschhorn syndrome and considerations regarding its correlation with other chromosomal disorders. Brain Dev 25: 283–7.
66. Zankl A, Addor MC, Maeder-Ingvar MM, et al. (2001) A characteristic EEG pattern in 4p-syndrome: Case report and review of the literature. Eur J Pediatr 160: 123–7.
67. Oksanen VE, Arvio MA, Peippo MM, et al. (2004) Temporo-occipital spikes: A typical EEG finding in Kabuki syndrome. Pediatr Neurol 30: 67–70.
68. Glaze D, Schultz RJ, Frost JD. (1998) Rett syndrome: Characterization of seizures versus non-seizures. Electroencephalogr Clin Neurophysiol 106: 79–83.
69. Koh S. Jayakar P, Dunoyer C, et al. (2000) Epilepsy surgery in children with tuberous sclerosis complex: Presurgical evaluation ond outcome. Epilepsia 41: 1206–13.
70. Kuzniecky RI. (2005) Neuroimaging of epilepsy: Therapeutic implications. NeuroRx. 2: 384–93.
71. ILAE Neuroimaging Comission. (1997) ILAE Neuroimaging commission recommendations for neuroimaging of patients with epilepsy. Epilepsia 38(Suppl. 10): 1–2.

Chapter 5
The Differential Diagnosis of Epilepsy

S. M. Zuberi

Introduction

Most children and adults seen in a first-seizure clinic or paroxysmal disorders clinic will not have epilepsy. There are as many, and likely many more, imitators and mimickers of epilepsy as there are different types of epileptic seizure. Several studies in adult and pediatric populations have shown high levels of misdiagnosis of epilepsy, consistently on the order of 25–50%[1, 2]. Unfortunately, the principal reason why many individuals are wrongly diagnosed is a lack of time and effort spent on the difficult art of history taking. In a first-seizure clinic the history takes clear precedence over the neurological examination, which in this context is often of limited value. Physicians must have an equally expert knowledge of the imitators of epilepsy as of the myriad clinical expressions of epileptic seizures in order to better refine and guide the history taking process.

The paramount importance of history taking is confirmed by the observation that misdiagnosis of epilepsy is high throughout the world, irrespective of the wealth and resources available to the health care system. Although the principal error is diagnosing epilepsy in an individual who does not have epileptic seizures, there are certain epileptic seizures, particularly those arising from the frontal lobe at nighttime, which may mimic nonepileptic events.[3]

The differential diagnosis of epilepsy encompasses the same spectrum of disorders and normal behaviors in individuals with and without intellectual disabilities (ID). In this context we must acknowledge that frequently any paroxysmal event in an individual with ID is often wrongly assumed to have an epileptic basis until proved otherwise. The physician must recognize that stereotypes and other behavioral events are more frequent and often more atypical in this population. A child or adult with a brain injury will have a higher risk of epileptic seizures than the general population. but they will also have a higher risk of nonepileptic myoclonus, sleep disturbance, and movement disorders. There are rare special situations leading to nonepileptic seizures, such as compulsive Valsalvas in children with autism resulting in anoxic seizures, which are rarely seen in the non-ID population. There are also many situations in which epileptic and nonepileptic disorders may coexist.

V.P. Prasher, M.P. Kerr (eds.) *Epilepsy and Intellectual Disabilities,*
DOI: 10.1007/978-1-84800-259-3_5, © Springer Science + Business Media, LLC 2008

The diagnosis of epilepsy must be positive and not based on exclusion of other possibilities. Evidence of an epileptic seizure from a detailed history should ideally be supported by additional investigations. If the physician is honest with the patients and caregivers concerning high levels of misdiagnosis, then it is unlikely they will begrudge the time taken to reach diagnostic certainty. There is often a perception that delaying the diagnosis of epilepsy will be dangerous and that doubt or uncertainty is a sign of a lack of the physician's skill. However, there is little evidence that reasonable delay in diagnosis is harmful. This compares to the mounting evidence that misdiagnosis leads to inappropriate medical treatments and limitation of educational and employment opportunities. If it is epilepsy, then continued review, an open mind, and the use of videotape recordings with or without electroencephalography (EEG) studies or ambulatory EEG may allow early diagnosis. For the individual with ID who requires respite or other community support, the diagnosis of an additional medical condition may result in withdrawal or limitation of support or an increased financial cost of that support. The impact of epilepsy misdiagnosis can span more than one generation; if a woman is inappropriately treated with medication through her pregnancy, her child is at risk from the teratogenic effects of antiepileptics, and the physician is at risk of a lawsuit.

In this chapter the term *seizure* is not synonymous with an event with an epileptic basis. Many terms such as *fit, seizure*, and *convulsion* are used interchangeably and can sometimes lead to confusion when ascribed to a particular individual. I believe it clarifies matters if we use the term *epileptic seizure* for a change in behavior caused by a hypersynchronous discharge of cortical neurons and use specific prefixes such as *pseudo-* or *psychogenic* or *nonepileptic* or *anoxic* when describing seizures that do not have an epileptic basis.

The diversity of nonepileptic events is considerable. Some of these nonepileptic events fully justify the term *nonepileptic seizure*.[4] The most common type of nonepileptic seizure leading to diagnostic confusion in clinical practice is the anoxic seizure, or syncopal convulsion.[5, 6]

When children suspected of having epilepsy are studied for diagnostic purposes in tertiary monitoring units, nonepileptic events predominate.[7, 8] In the study of Bye and colleagues,[7] which included children with ID, psychological and sleep phenomena were most common, and the EEG frequently showed misleading "epileptiform" discharges. Kotagal and colleagues[8] reported on 134 children and adolescents referred to a pediatric epilepsy monitoring unit at the Cleveland Clinic over a 6-year period. They divided their results into three age groups. In the preschool, two-month to five-year group, the most common diagnoses were stereotypies, sleep jerks, parasomnias, and Sandifer syndrome. In the school-age 5- to 12-year group the most common diagnoses were conversion disorder (psychogenic pseudoepileptic seizures), inattention or day dreaming, stereotypies, sleep jerks, and paroxysmal movement disorders. In the adolescent 12- to 18-year group, over 80% had a diagnosis of conversion disorder (hysteria, psychogenic pseudoepileptic seizures). A significant proportion, 19–46%, of the children studied had concomitant epilepsy.

Classification of Nonepileptic Seizures and Events

Nonepileptic seizures and events can be classified into six broad and sometimes overlapping clinical categories:

1. Syncopes and anoxic seizures.
2. Psychological disorders.
3. Derangements of the sleep process.
4. Paroxysmal movement disorders.
5. Migraine and disorders possibly related to migraine.
6. Miscellaneous neurological events.

Syncopes and Anoxic Seizures

The term *anoxic seizure* is shorthand for the clinical or electroclinical event that occurs as a result of the cessation of nutrition to the most metabolically active neurons. The anoxic seizure is the consequence of a syncope, that is, the abrupt cutting off of the energy substrates to the cerebral cortex, usually through a sudden decrease in cerebral perfusion by oxygenated blood. Less complete or less rapidly evolving syncopes have less dramatic consequences. The seizure may manifest as a mixture of sensory symptoms, jerks, stiffening, and altered consciousness.

Although I have divided the syncopes into various categories, considerable overlap occurs. In particular, it seems likely that vasovagal syncope, neurocardiogenic syncope, reflex anoxic seizures or reflex asystolic syncope (RAS), and breath-holding spells or prolonged expiratory apnea are all varieties of neurally mediated syncope. When adults, caregivers, parents, or children require more information or are upset when told that it's only breath holding or only a simple faint, contact with an organization which provides support and additional literature may be very helpful (http://www.stars.org.uk).

Reflex Anoxic Seizures or Reflex Asystolic Syncope: RAS

Gastaut used the term reflex anoxic cerebral seizures to describe all the various syncopes, sobbing spasms, and breath-holding spells that followed noxious stimuli in young children.[9] Since 1978, reflex anoxic seizure has been used more specifically to describe a particular type of nonepileptic convulsive event, most commonly induced in young children by an unexpected bump to the head.[10] Although other terminology, such as pallid/white breath-holding and pallid infantile syncope, has been applied to such episodes, the term reflex anoxic seizure is now widely recognized. More recently, the term reflex asystolic syncope has been used. Until the advent of cardiac loop recorders, direct evidence with respect to the pathophysiology of natural attacks has been very limited. Since prolonged cardiac recording has become feasible in children, many recordings of prolonged reflex asystole have been recorded and several examples published.[11,12]

A typical history would be that of a child who in response to a bump on the head or a cut will go "white as a sheet," lose consciousness, and then collapse to the floor, sometimes becoming floppy and then recovering but frequently progressing to dystonic extension of limbs and a few irregular spasms or jerks of the body. The loss of consciousness, collapse, stiffenings, and jerking movements are the anoxic seizure. The abnormal movements are brainstem release phenomena and are not epileptic in origin. They occur because the syncope has cut off nutrition to the higher centers of the cerebral cortex.

The caregivers will be terrified, often believing the child has died. The child may recover consciousness rapidly, within seconds, but may be miserable and tired, and some children continue to sleep for an hour or more. Although the "seizure" may last seconds, the caregiver's perception will be that it has lasted for minutes. Using the second hand of a watch while the witness tries to replay the image in their mind's eye will often help to differentiate between seconds and minutes.

As children grow older, reflex anoxic seizures may cease altogether or change to more obvious convulsive or nonconvulsive vasovagal syncope in childhood and adolescence. It is possible, although proper long-term studies have not been done, that syncopes may reappear in old age.

Beyond the toddler stage, individuals may report sensory disturbances along with the syncopes. Most dramatic are out-of-body experiences with a dream-like quality, which may include the feeling of having floated up to the ceiling and and watching his or her body lying on the floor in a seizure.[13] Night terrors (see *"pavor nocturnus"* below) as a sequel to the syncopal episodes have also been reported by parents.

It is best to try to make a precise diagnosis as to whether a convulsive syncope in a young child is cardiogenic or respiratory in origin. If it is cardiogenic, then the main differential diagnosis is a reflex anoxic seizure (reflex asystolic syncope) versus a convulsive syncope from long QT syndrome or other cardiac cause. If it appears to be a respiratory (i.e., apneic) syncope, then the differential diagnosis is breath-holding spells (prolonged end-expiratory apnea) or suffocation, in particular from imposed upper airway obstruction.

Vasovagal Syncope

Vasovagal syncope is the most familiar and predominant form of neurally mediated syncope. If classic reflex anoxic seizures (with reflex asystolic syncope) represent a fairly pure vagal attack, vasovagal syncope involves a vasodepressor component with variable vagal accompaniment. Episodes may begin in infancy, sometimes with reflex anoxic seizures, and thereafter are seen at all ages, becoming most dramatic perhaps in old age.[14]

Tables in medical textbooks or works of epileptology tend to perpetuate gross errors with respect to the distinction between vasovagal syncope and comparable epileptic seizures. This may be in part because many authors equate syncope with some sort of limp pallid swooning in the Victorian manner. Features mistakenly used to distinguish syncope and epileptic seizures have included incontinence, postictal sleep, injury, and convulsive jerks. In reality the situation is different. Vasovagal syncope may occur supine, particularly in the case of venipuncture fits, though some would call these reflex anoxic seizures, as the mechanism is strongly cardioinhibitory. Pallor and sweating are certainly not invariable, nor need onset be gradual. There is no difference between the liability to injury in convulsive syncope as opposed to a comparable convulsive epileptic seizure. Convulsive jerks are certainly not rare but occur in perhaps 50% of vasovagal syncopes and more often in experimental syncope.[15] Urinary incontinence is common, occurring in 10% of cases in one experimental study.[16] Unconsciousness may be much more than seconds and recovery, although it may be rapid in mild syncope, is not necessarily complete early on. It is true that postictal confusion, proper, is rare, but it can occur. Vasovagal syncope can occur more than once per day. Stimuli maybe very subtle, but it's true that some sort of stimulus should be detected for at least some attacks in any individual.

The setting and stimulus are indeed the most important factors in allowing the presumptive diagnosis of vasovagal syncope, together with elicitation of the warning symptoms or aura, which are commonly present. A seizure which occurs while the individual's hair is being blow-dried or brushed is almost always a vasovagal nonepileptic convulsive syncope. Premonitory symptoms are usually present even if the duration is only a second or two, but sometimes these are forgotten and only recalled when syncope is reproduced, as in the head-up tilt test. All physicians are aware of the usual symptoms of cerebral ischemia, such as dizziness and greying out of vision and tinnitus, but an important additional symptom is abdominal pain. It may be difficult to tell whether abdominal pain is a symptom or trigger of a vasovagal syncope or an intestinal symptom of a strong vagal discharge. The latter is quite common and sometimes leads to confusion with the epigastic aura which may precede the complex partial component of a temporal lobe epileptic seizure. Almost all individuals with vasovagal syncope have a first-degree relative, commonly a parent, affected.[17] Sometimes this leads to more than one generation of a family being misdiagnosed as having epilepsy.

Occasionally head-up tilt testing may be useful not only as a diagnostic aid but as a diagnostic reinforcer. If everyone is convinced that the individual with convulsive syncope has "grand mal" epilepsy then reproducing the event on a tilt table may be helpful in undoing the wrong diagnosis. The test must reproduce the typical event. It must be remembered that an individual with epilepsy may also faint or have a drop in blood pressure during a tilt test.

Vagovagal Syncope

By contrast to vasovagal syncope, convincing vagovagal syncope is rare. The reflex is usually triggered by swallowing or vomiting; cardiac standstill results if the asystole is sufficiently prolonged, with a convulsive syncope (anoxic seizure). This is probably not a life-threatening disorder, but the symptoms can be troublesome, particularly if the patient also has migraine with associated vomiting. Pacemaker therapy can be considered if events are frequent and interfering with quality of life.

Hyperventilation Syncope

Hyperventilation in any human induces various organic symptoms which may in certain individuals stimulate further hyperventilation and exacerbation of the original symptoms. A degree of panic may be so engendered. Hyperventilation in the clinic may reproduce the concerning symptoms.

Hyperventilation may trigger both epileptic and nonepileptic absences.[18]

Individuals with Rett syndrome may have hyperventilation, apnea, complex behavioral stereotypies, and epileptic seizures, which may lead to diagnostic and therapeutic difficulties.

Orthostasis

Syncope due to orthostatic hypotension secondary to autonomic failure is uncommon. Dopamine ß-decarboxylase deficiency is a possibility in such a clinical situation.[19] The simplest way of detecting orthostatic intolerance is to stand the individual on a foam mat (to avoid injury when falling) for 10 minutes with continuous blood pressure measurements. This method may also be used to provoke vasovagal syncope in young children, including those too young to tilt.[20]

Chronic orthostatic intolerance can produce other symptoms, including symptoms of presyncope: lightheadedness, "dizziness," and blurred vision. Furthermore, exercise intolerance, chronic fatigue, migrainous headache, nausea, abdominal discomfort, chest discomfort, palpitations, shortness of breath, hyperventilation, peripheral cyanosis, and sweating and flushing on standing have been described in this condition.[21]

Chronic orthostatic intolerance is sometimes part of the clinical picture in chronic fatigue syndromes, and it maybe helpful to consider this treatable disorder as a differential of idiopathic chronic fatigue syndrome.

One clinical picture comprising chronic orthostatic intolerance in teenagers and young adults is the postural orthostatic tachycardia syndrome (POTS).[22] Patients have symptoms of chronic orthostatic intolerance with significant daily disability associated with a marked tachycardia on standing: a heart rate increase of >30 beats/minute or a heart rate of >120 beats/minute within 10 minutes of head-up tilt.[21]

Long QT Disorders

The long QT syndromes are associated with genuinely life-threatening syncopes, which may be hypotonic or convulsive. The mechanism of the syncopes is a ventricular tachyarrhythmia, normally torsades de pointes. As a rule, there is no great difficulty in the diagnosis of the syndrome of Jervell and Lange-Nielsen, in which congenital deafness is associated with an autosomal recessive inheritance.[23] Much more difficult is the Romano-Ward syndrome, which is dominantly inherited but with incomplete penetrance. There is a degree of overlap between the stimuli which induce the neurally mediated syncopes and those which trigger the ventricular tachyarrhythmias of the long QT syndrome. The two situations in which cardiac arrhythmias have to be actively considered are those in which convulsions occur:

1. During exercise, especially when that exercise is emotionally charged;
2. Events triggered by fear or fright.

Long QT disorders are very much less common than neurally mediated syncopes such as reflex anoxic seizures/reflex asystolic syncope, but this diagnosis should be sought when the precipitants of a cardiac syncope are not of the typical benign reflex anoxic seizure type (that is to say unexpected bumps to the head). This is another reason for trying to separate by history cardiac and respiratory syncopes.

A child was recently referred to the neurology service in our hospital with a history of convulsions triggered by fear or fright such as "*seeing a mask at a Halloween party.*" This, along with the history contained in the referral letter that the boy had a cochlear implant, was enough for us to expedite the appointment, arrange an electrocardiogram (ECG) rather than an EEG, and refer to the cardiology department. It must be remembered that in the same way that an interictal EEG may be normal in a child with epilepsy, a brief 12-lead ECG may be normal in a child with cardiac arrhythmias. If the diagnosis is strongly suspected, a referral to cardiology is appropriate even with a normal ECG.

Long QT syndrome and other cardiac arrhythmias such as short QT syndrome may result in sudden death. Treatment is in the realm of cardiology but may include beta blockers and implantable defibrillators.

Long QT syndromes are principally caused by mutations in ion channel genes, as are the majority of the idiopathic epilepsies. It is reasonable to think of cardiac arrhythmias as epilepsies of the heart and epilepsies as recurrent arrhythmias of the brain.[24]

Breath-Holding Attacks

Breath-holding spells have been described for centuries, but controversy as to what they are remains.[25, 26] The term *breath-holding* is not at all satisfactory.[27] It tends to give offense to parents of affected children. It seems to imply temper tantrums and bad behavior. In some pediatric textbooks breath-holding attacks are to be found in the section on psychiatric or psychological disorders. However, studies have shown that however one defines breath-holding spells, behavioral disorders in those afflicted do not differ from those in control children.[28]

Breath-holding seems to imply some sort of voluntary "I'll hold my breath until I get what I want" behavior, but this is not correct. There is no difficulty nowadays in recognizing that what used to be called white or pallid breath-holding has a cardiac rather than a respiratory mechanism, as discussed earlier in the section on reflex anoxic seizures/reflex asystolic syncope. The term *prolonged expiratory apnea* is certainly helpful in discussing those episodes in which the mechanism is predominantly respiratory, even though the pathophysiological details may be in dispute.[29]

Very few polygraphic recordings of children have been made. There appears to be a pure respiratory "breath-holding" spell or prolonged expiratory apnea, without any change in cardiac rate or rhythm (albeit information on cardiac output is not available), such attacks being clearly cyanotic or "blue" breath-holding. The expiratory apnea is frequently silent but sometimes accompanied by small grunts in association with the series of small expirations. The child becomes cyanosed, loses consciousness followed by secondary anoxic seizure characterized by stiffening, often decerebrate in appearance, and a few irregular jerks of the limbs. As in RAS there may be a rapid recovery or more prolonged sleepiness. There are also episodes which may be described as "mixed" breath-holding in so far as not only is there expiratory apnea but also a degree of bradycardia or cardiac asystole.[4]

The key aspect of management is reassurance and prevention of the diagnosis of epilepsy. The use of iron therapy has been suggested in children who have iron deficiency anemia.[30]

Compulsive Valsalva

Children with ID, including those with autistic disorders, may self-induce syncopes resulting in atonic or convulsive anoxic seizures. This may prove a major diagnostic challenge, as epilepsy may also occur in these individuals. Many seizures in Rett syndrome may be the result of self-induced syncopes.[31] The mechanisms are very much like the experimental syncopes described by Lempert and colleagues.[15] Diagnosis may only be possible with careful viewing of videotape recordings of the event or detailed polygraphic recordings. These individuals may hyperventilate and then hold their breath in inspiration. If they go on to do a Valsalva with a closed glottis they will effectively obstruct the cerebral circulation. If this persists for more than 5–10 seconds, an anoxic seizure will result. These events are termed compulsive Valsalvas and may become frequent. The individual may be getting a pleasurable experience from the presyncope or syncopal experience, leading to reinforcement of the behavior.[32] Such episodes may be very severe and, indeed, may have a fatal outcome.[33] The syncope produced by a compulsive Valsalva may be one of the situations where reduced cerebral perfusion and hypoxia may trigger a secondary epileptic seizure — the anoxic-epileptic seizure. These anoxic-epileptic seizures are frequently prolonged, resulting in status epilepticus and the requirement for rescue medication.[34] The epileptic component can be differentiated from the syncope and anoxic seizure because of its nature and duration. Videotape recordings are once again very helpful in unraveling this complex situation.

If secondary epileptic seizures are frequent, antiepileptic medication may be justified. This may prevent the epileptic component but not the syncope or anoxic seizure. Anoxic-epileptic seizures may follow on from any syncope including RAS and breath-holding.[34]

Psychological Disorders

Some of the disorders listed in this section may not be fundamentally different from some of the other disorders here described, particularly in the sections on vasovagal syncope and hyperventilation syncope above, but what are often called psychological mechanisms seem of more obvious importance here.

Daydreams

There is general awareness of episodes referred to as daydreams, which may be mistaken for epileptic or anoxic (syncopal) absences. There may not be a fundamental difference from that described in the next subsection as gratification, but the subsequent conditions are more likely to lead to diagnostic difficulties, as abnormal movements are more prominent. Time-out periods or daydreams are seen more frequently in individuals with specific and general learning disability. Observers are often adamant that they cannot distract an individual from an event. This is not a useful distinguishing feature compared to seeking the positive features of epileptic absences, including eye flickering and subtle loss of muscle tone. Epileptic absences are brief, usually lasting seconds, and usually occur more frequently than daydreams. The distinction in individuals with learning disability, particularly in those who may already have a diagnosis of epilepsy, is not always straightforward and may require ambulatory EEG monitoring to show that the staring episodes are not epileptic.

Gratification and Stereotypies

More or less pleasurable behavior, apparently similar to masturbation, may be seen from infancy onwards, more so in preschool girls. Rhythmic hip flexion and adduction may be accompanied by a distant expression and perhaps somnolence thereafter. Manual stimulation of the genitalia does not seem necessary. Sometimes the prominent feature is dystonic extension of the lower limbs.[35] The diagnosis of infantile masturbation is more difficult when the infant or young child seems unhappy during the rhythmic movements. The relative frequency of events and occurrence in specific circumstances, such as when bored or in a car seat or high chair, lends this behavior to home videotape recording. Parents prefer the term gratification to infantile masturbation, understandably.

Hand flapping, finger sucking, head banging, and body rocking stereotypies are more common in individuals with pervasive developmental disorders with or without global learning disability than in the ID population.[36] They often occur in response to excitement but may also be regarded as a form of self-stimulation. More complex stereotypies, such as repetitive finger movements, rotation of the hands and wrists, and head thrusting and body flexing behaviors may be difficult to distinguish from complex tics. Videotape analysis is key to the diagnosis. I have seen several videotapes of complex stereotypies and gratification misdiagnosed as paroxysmal dyskinesia, which has led to inappropriate therapy with carbamazepine.

Sometimes more difficult to diagnose may be the phenomenon in slightly older children, of the "television in the sky," or eidetic imagery. Affected children may appear to stare into space or have unvocalized speech with imaginary individuals and perhaps seem to twitch or move one or more limbs for several minutes at a time. When there are repeated jerks or spasms, there may be confusion with epileptic infantile spasms or focal epileptic seizure with impairment of awareness.

Out-of-Body Experiences

There are several situations in which individuals may describe experiences in which they appear to lose immediate contact with their bodies and perhaps see themselves from above. Such hallucinations and dissociative states have been described in epileptic seizures, anoxic seizures, migraine, and as a "normal" phenomenon.[37,38] Some of these perceptual disorders may be described as the "Alice in Wonderland phenomenon."

Panic/Anxiety

Panic attacks are well recognized in adults and children and have been well reviewed.[39] However, it is important to recognize that panic attacks may actually be manifestations of epileptic seizures.[40,41] Long-term video-EEG monitoring may be necessary to establish the correct diagnosis and prevent inappropriate psychiatric interventions.

Conversion Disorder

Whether the term hysteria should be used is debated, but self-induced nonepileptic, nonsyncopal seizures are not rare.[8] Such episodes are called various names, such as "pseudoseizures," "pseudoepileptic seizures," "psychogenic nonepileptic seizures," "nonepileptic attack disorder," or "emotional attacks"; none of these terms are satisfactory for every case. The episodes may crudely mimic epileptic seizures and have some resemblance to certain frontal lobe epileptic seizures but often have prominent sexual and aggressive components. They are usually recognized readily by observation and particularly by videotape observation and do not include alteration in background EEG. Some are predominantly swoons: a more or less graceful collapse without injury often into a recovery position, in some rhythmic jerking of the head, one or more limbs or trunk or thrusting of the pelvis predominates. Rolling from side to side with eyes closed is often seen, a feature not characteristic of an epileptic seizure. Rapid symmetrical jerking may stop suddenly in contrast to the gradual slowing in frequency seen in a generalized clonic epileptic seizure. In some cases incest, sexual abuse, or other cause of posttraumatic stress disorder may be the etiology.[42,43] The possibility of nonepileptic seizures in an individual with true epilepsy has to be considered when the seizure type or frequency changes unexpectedly.

"Psychosomatic" syncope has been described in adults who collapse on head-up tilt with normal vital signs.[44] Collapse occurs without change in heart rate, blood pressure, or EEG. The differential diagnosis here includes hyperventilation syncope (see above).

The psychiatric literature has changed terms over the years, from hysteria to conversion hysteria to conversion disorders to dissociative states, without adding precision or clarity. A sociomedical model is useful for professionals: considering the illness "real" while recognizing that it may be an inevitable response to a particular "predicament" and allowing the patient to recover while saving face.[45,46] We strongly recommend to readers a clear and modern view of hysteria.[47]

Reassurance and encouragement, with or without simple behavioral techniques, will often work; however, in difficult cases psychiatric management will need to be available.

Derangments of the Sleep Process

While it is certain that all the funny turns which may occur in the daytime have not yet been properly described in the literature, it is even more likely that the disorders of the sleep process are by no means fully described. There are great intrinsic difficulties in readily determining what happens during sleep. Even ordinary visual observation may be difficult, whereas videorecording and, even more, polygraphic recording, may only be possible in exceptional cases where episodes are very frequent. It is important to recognize that all parasomnias have not yet been described and to question carefully the origin of any episode which occurs only during sleep, even though some disorders previously thought to be parasomnias have now been found to be epileptic.[3]

The parasomnias and neurological sleep disorders such as narcolepsy may be confused with epilepsy due to their paroxysmal nature. The difficulties in distinguishing epileptic and nonepileptic events is compounded by the fact that paroxysmal nonepileptic sleep events are more common in children with epilepsy or ID than in the general childhood population. Sleep disorders remain a largely neglected and poorly understood area in pediatrics; however, with careful attention to the timing and semiology of events and the use of video EEG and nocturnal polysomnography these conditions can be classified and differentiated from epileptic seizures.

Parasomnias

A detailed history will distinguish most parasomnias from epileptic seizures. Parasomnias typically occur only once or twice a night. If events are occurring at a frequency of three or more times a night, the strong likelihood is that they are epileptic in nature, most likely arising from mesial/orbital frontal lobe structures. Epileptic seizures tend to occur more frequently in stage II sleep but may occur throughout sleep. In differentiating these events video polysomnography is the most useful investigative tool. Recently a clinical scoring scale has been devised to try and help distinguish parasomnias and nocturnal frontal lobe epilepsy.[48]

Non-REM Partial Arousal Disorders/Arousal Parasomnias/Night Terrors

Brief nocturnal arousals are normal in children and adults. They occur typically in stage IV non-REM sleep disorders, one to two hours after sleep onset. They vary from normal events such as mumbling, chewing, sitting up, and staring to arousals which can be thought of as abnormal because of the disruption they cause the family. There is frequently a family history of parasomnias, and although non-REM partial arousals / Arsoual parasomnias / Night terrors are primarily a problem of childhood they may persist into adult life. These include calm and agitated sleepwalking, and a spectrum from confusional arousals to night terrors or *pavor nocturnes*.[49] The individual may exhibit automatic behavior, but the events are not truly stereotyped. Affected children may be very agitated and look frightened, as if they do not recognize their parents. They are in an intermediate stage between waking and sleep, so they may respond, but not normally. They look awake and may be partially responsive but in fact are still in deep slow-wave sleep (stage IV). These events typically only occur once a night, especially one or two hours after falling asleep and nearly always in the first half of sleep. Children have no memory of them. Often they are very prolonged, and it is 10 to 15 minutes before the child either wakes or settles back to restful sleep. By contrast, nocturnal frontal lobe epileptic seizures typically last less than two minutes and will often occur in clusters.

The distinction between NREM arousal disorders and benign partial epilepsy with affective symptoms (BPEAS), a variety of idiopathic focal epilepsy like benign Rolandic epilepsy, can be more difficult.[50] Children arouse and look similarly wild and combative. The epileptic seizures are, however, brief, and may occur while awake and in sleep; they do not arise particularly from stage IV sleep and are more likely to occur towards the end of sleep, in the early morning. NREM arousal disorders likely represent a disordered balance between the drive to wake and the drive to sleep. They are more common in toddlers who sleep very deeply, in children who are overtired because of insufficient sleep, and those who are unwell or on certain medications. An increased drive to wake occurs if the child has an irregular sleep schedule, is unwell, or needs environmental associations to fall asleep normally. These disorders are therefore primarily managed by reassurance, explanation, and behavioral means measures to establish stable sleep routines and ensure good sleep hygiene. Home videotape recording is invaluable, particularly if the camera can be left running to capture the onset of the event. It is generally true that home videotape of nocturnal events is more likely to be successful if the seizures are nocturnal frontal lobe rather than partial arousals due to the relative frequency and clustering of epileptic events.

REM Sleep Disorders

Nightmares and sleep paralysis are the principal REM sleep disorders that may be confused with epilepsy. They are both common. Ten percent to 20% of individuals will have some experience of sleep paralysis. Waking from REM sleep without abolishing the physiological REM atonia that prevents us from "acting out" our dreams may lead to a frightening experience of paralysis. Nightmares are usually easier to distinguish from epileptic seizures than night terrors, as the child will have a memory of both waking and of the dream, and will then move into normal wakefulness rapidly. Nocturnal epileptic seizures rarely arise out of REM sleep.

Behavioral management and treatment of any comorbid medical conditions are the appropriate treatment strategies. The onset of a REM behavior disorder may rarely be the first clinical sign of a brainstem lesion, and neuroimaging may be appropriate. In adults REM behavior disorders and acting out of dreams, sometimes violent, may predate by many years other symptoms of serious neurological disorders such as Parkinsons disease, dementia with Lewy bodies, or multiple system atrophy.[51]

Sleep-Wake Transition Disorders

Head Banging and Body Rocking

Rhythmic movement disorders such as nocturnal head banging (*jactatio capitis nocturna*), body rocking, and head rolling typically occur in infants and toddlers as they are trying to fall asleep. They can be present in deep sleep and in wakefulness. They are more common in children with ID. They will typically remit by five years of age but may persist into adult life. Management relies on good sleep hygiene and padding the headboard so the rest of the house is not awakened. Rhythmic movement disorders that are not clearly associated with the sleep-wake transition state but persist through the night respond less well to behavioral management techniques; rarely, medications such as benzodiazepines may be helpful. There are occasional reports of head banging in adults.[52]

Sleep Starts/Hypnic Jerks

Vigevano's group used videorecordings to report repetitive sleep starts in children who also had epilepsy and tetraplegic cerebral palsy.[53] These jerks occurred repetitively at the onset of sleep in clusters lasting several minutes, with arousal appearance on EEG but no jerk-related spike discharges. The authors emphasized the need to differentiate these sleep starts from epileptic seizures, particularly as the children also had epilepsy, so as to avoid excessive inappropriate antiepileptic medication. I have had personal experience of a child with Down syndrome who had recovered from West syndrome but presented for reevaluation of seizures in sleep. These proved to be sleep starts.

The Narcolepsy-Cataplexy Syndrome

Narcolepsy is a disorder characterized by excessive daytime sleepiness, cataplexy (a loss of tone in response to strong emotion, typically laughter), sleep paralysis, hypnagogic hallucinations, and disturbed nighttime sleep. A third of adults describe onset before 16 years of age, about 16% before 10 years of age, and around 4% less than 5 years.[54] Consciousness is maintained during cataplexy even though the eyes may be closed. Typically the loss of tone spreads from the face down the body. The individual has a degree of control, so as they collapse this often appears to occur in a series of stages rather than a sudden fall. In six children I diagnosed with narcolepsy between 1997 and 2000, four previously had been given a diagnosis of epilepsy: either "absences" because of the excessive sleepiness, myoclonic drop attacks because of the cataplexy, or partial seizures because the cataplexy was asymmetric. One child had been treated with multiple antiepileptic medications.[55] Diagnosis rests on recognition of the five features of the syndrome, videorecording of cataplexy, if possible and if practicable, and the multiple sleep latency test, provided the child is years old or older.[56]

Paroxysmal Movement Disorders

There is a complex relationship between epilepsy and movement disorders, the boundaries of which are difficult to define.[57] They share many symptoms and are frequently confused with each other. Paroxysmal movement disorders are characterized by variable duration of motor symptoms, usually with few if any interictal abnormalities on examination. Some children with "intermediate" exertion-related dystonia have subtle dystonia or signs of developmental dyspraxia, even on good days. The major distinguishing features between these events and epileptic seizures are the frequent presence of precipitating factors and the retention of consciousness in the paroxysmal dyskinesias and ataxias. These features may be more difficult to determine in childhood.

Paroxysmal Dyskinesias

Various complex classifications have been proposed for this group of disorders.[58] The most clinically relevant and simplest is used below. Most of the literature describes familial cases which are easier to diagnose (especially once one or more affected family members are known) and are possibly more interesting to report than sporadic cases. However, clinical experience suggests that most cases are sporadic and that many do not fit exactly into the classic descriptions outlined below.

Paroxysmal Kinesigenic Dyskinesia (PKD)

Typically, onset is in early childhood or adolescence with brief episodes of choreoathetosis, dystonia, or a mixed pattern. Attacks tend to become less frequent or remit totally in adult life. Attacks last seconds to five minutes and are precipitated by sudden movements, change in position, or change in movement velocity.[59] Getting up from a chair or getting out of a car frequently trigger attacks. Consciousness is retained, and some individuals may have a brief nonspecific warning or aura prior to an attack. Interictal examination is normal. Diagnosis is based on history, and a videorecording of events is invaluable. Carbamazepine is often highly effective in small doses. There is a family history of similar events in about a quarter of patients with autosomal dominant inheritance in many families.

Paroxysmal Nonkinesigenic Dyskinesia (PNKD)

Attacks are often longer in PNKD and may last two minutes to several hours or even two days. This type is sometimes referred to as paroxysmal dystonic choreoathetosis (PDC). The attacks are often markedly dystonic and occur spontaneously, though in adults alcohol, caffeine, and stress are frequent precipitants. Differentiation from epileptic seizures is easier, and treatment with antiepileptic medications is less effective. Inheritance is usually autosomal dominant.

Paroxysmal Exercise-Induced Dyskinesia (PED)

Events occur after several minutes of exercise, usually 10–15 minutes or more, not at the initiation of movement as in PKD.[59] Typically, the part of the body that has been doing most exercise will become dystonic. The abnormal movement will resolve gradually, with cessation of the exercise over 5–30 minutes (intermediate between PKC and classic PDC). Antiepileptic medications are not generally helpful, though acetazolamide has been effective in some families.[60]

Episodic Ataxias

Episodic ataxia type 1 (EA1) is a rare disorder caused by mutations in a voltage-gated potassium channel Kv1.1. Affected individuals have brief episodes of cerebellar ataxia lasting seconds or minutes.[61] The episodes are triggered by sudden movement, exercise, stress, or emotion. Sometimes the movement disorder appears more like dystonia or choreoathetosis rather than ataxia. Interictal myokymia, detected clinically by observation of fine finger movements or rippling eyelid muscles, or by demonstration of continuous motor unit activity on EMG, is the principal diagnostic feature. In addition to paroxysmal ataxia being confused with a partial epileptic seizure there is a real overrepresentation of epilepsy in families with EA1.[62,63]

Migraine and Disorders Possibly Related to Migraine

Some authors regard migraine with aura as an important differential in the diagnosis of epilepsy.[64] There are a number of conditions ranging from undoubted varieties of definite migraine through migraine equivalents probably having a migrainous origin to conditions in which the migraine link is more tenuous. On the whole, the more classic the migraine picture, the easier the diagnosis.

Familial Hemiplegic Migraine

Since virtually all attacks of familial hemiplegic migraine (FHM) are associated with headache and a family history of hemiplegic migraine, the differential diagnosis should not normally be difficult.[65] The hemiplegia occurs during the aura phase of the migraine.

Benign Paroxysmal Vertigo of Childhood

This is the most common of the migraine equivalents.[66] Although affected pre-school children are often referred as patients with epilepsy, the characteristic history of anxious arrest of movement without loss of awareness and subjective vertigo, or "drunking," makes the diagnosis easy.

Alternating Hemiplegia

The paroxysmal features and neurology of alternating hemiplegia of childhood are remarkable and fascinating. In their original report Verret and Steele described eight cases from the Hospital for Sick Children, Toronto; they regarded the condition as infantile-onset complicated migraine.[67] Most recently, 44 patients were reported from Boston.[68] These and other figures suggest that the condition has in the past been both underdiagnosed and underreported.

Attacks of flaccid hemiplegia on one or other, or both sides, begin in the first 18 months of life and are associated with autonomic phenomena and the gradual appearance of developmental delay unsteadiness and a degree of choreoathetosis. The first hemiplegic attack is not usually noticed until after the age of six months. The initial manifestations often begin in the neonatal period with tonic and dystonic attacks and a disorder of eye movement, in particular paroxysmal, often unilateral, nystagmus and strabismus. There may be transitory internuclear ophthalmoplegia.[69] Pallor, crying, screaming, or general misery accompany these attacks.

Miscellaneous Neurologic Events

There are many paroxysmal disorders which are of neurologic origin and which may be mistaken for epileptic seizures but which do not easily fit into the classification described. Many of them are specific to certain genetic syndromes. It is not possible to give a complete picture — many types of event, convulsion, fit, seizure, attack, turn, spell, or whatever have yet to be described.

Tics

Brief, sudden, irregularly occurring movements or sounds are common. The subjective urge to produce the movement and a degree of suppressibility are the keys to the diagnosis of tics. In individuals with learning disability these features may not be as easily identified, and the alternative diagnosis of an epileptic origin may be determined by recording an EEG during the tic, preferably with simultaneous videorecording.

Myoclonus

Nonepileptic myoclonus occurs in many situations. It is common in situations where there is reduced cortical inhibition of brainstem and spinal reflexes, for example in various types of cerebral palsy or congenital microcephaly. If there is difficulty in diagnosis, EEG will determine whether the myoclonus is epileptic or not. The EEG (preferably with surface EMG and videorecording simultaneously) will show obvious spike discharges during epileptic myoclonus.

Cataplexy in Neurologic Disorders

Cataplexy in the narcolepsy-cataplexy syndrome has been discussed in "Derangements of the Sleep Process." Cataplexy is rarely associated with acquired brainstem lesions, such as occur in multiple sclerosis. Cataplexy may be seen in Niemann-Pick type C, Norrie disease, the Prader-Willi syndrome, and as an isolated familial trait.[70] Recognition is based on the identification of emotional triggers, especially laughter, to the sudden loss of muscle tone.

Coffin-Lowry Syndrome

Early reports suggested that epilepsy was a feature of the X-linked but female-manifesting Coffin-Lowry syndrome (CLS). Later publications, including a series from our center, suggested that those with CLS did not have epilepsy but a cataplexy-like disorder, triggered by the startle effect of unexpected sounds and the emotion of laughter.[71] We have reported that reflex stiffenings, loss of tone with emotion ("cataplexy"), and epileptic seizures may occur in a single individual.[72]

Movement Disorders of Glut-1-Deficiency Syndrome

It is important for physicians to recognize that impaired glucose transport across the blood-brain barrier results in Glut-1-deficiency syndrome. Classic cases are characterized by infantile seizures, developmental delay, acquired microcephaly, ataxia, and hypoglycorrhachia.[73] As expected, in this relatively recently described genetic disorder, the associated phenotype is expanding. It includes individuals with mild or no learning disability, normal head circumference, and paroxysmal movement abnormalities such as ataxia, dystonia, and choreoathetosis. Diagnosis is based on finding an inappropriately low fasting CSF glucose (typical CSF:blood glucose <0.4). This disorder can be treated effectively by providing the brain with an alternative fuel through the ketogenic diet.

Conclusion

A precise, detailed, all-embracing history remains paramount in correctly recognizing the paroxysmal disorders that make up the differential diagnosis of epilepsy in individuals with or without learning disability. Sufficient time needs to be set aside for the history and strenuous efforts made to speak first hand to witnesses. Home videorecording is an invaluable tool, and physicians should not be slow in requesting video-EEG telemetry if this will aid in preventing misdiagnosis. Every paroxysmal disorders/epilepsy clinic should have facilities for viewing videorecordings in a variety of formats. Epileptic and nonepileptic seizures can coexist in this population. When individuals, even with definite epilepsy, have a new type of event or increasing seizures not responsive to medication, the diagnosis must be critically reviewed.

The physician must not be afraid to ask for further opinions. This process is aided by technology which allows digital copying of videos to CD and computer files. It is a truism but worthwhile repeating that we often only recognize medical disorders that we have seen and diagnosed previously. Families and caregivers should be encouraged to bring videorecordings to the clinic and asked if they will consent, with appropriate safeguards, to the video being shown to other families and health workers. The *"That's it!"* phenomenon is an important technique for both caregivers and professionals.

References

1. Udall, P, Alving J, Hansen LK, et al. (2006) The misdiagnosis of epilepsy in children admitted to a tertiary epilepsy centre with paroxysmal events. Arch Dis Child 91:219–21.
2. Ferrie CD. (2006) Preventing misdiagnosis of epilepsy. Arch Dis Child 91:206–9.
3. Scheffer IE, Bhatia KP, Lopes Cendes I, et al. (1994) Autosomal dominant nocturnal frontal lobe epilepsy diagnosed as a sleep disorder. Lancet 343:515–17.
4. Stephenson JBP. (1990) Fits and faints. Cambridge and New York: MacKeith Press and Cambridge University Press.
5. Stephenson JBP. (2001) Anoxic seizures: Self-terminating syncopes. Epileptic Disord 3: 3–6.
6. Smith PE, Myson V, Gibbon F. (2002) A teenage epilepsy clinic: Observational study. Eur J Neurol 9: 373–6.
7. Bye AM, Kok DJ, Ferenschild FT, et al. (2000) Paroxysmal non-epileptic events in children: A retrospective study over a period of 10 years. J Pediatr Child Health 36: 244–8.
8. Kotagal P, Costa M, Wyllie E, et al. (2002) Paroxysmal non-epileptic events in children and adolescence. Pediatrics 110: E46.
9. Gastaut H. (1968) Aphysiopathogenic study of reflex anoxic cerebral sizures in children (syncopes, sobbing spasms and breath holding spells). In Kellaway P, Petersen I (eds.). Clinical electroencephalography of children. Stockholm: Almquist and Wiksell.
10. Stephenson JBP. (1978) Two types of febrile seizure-anoxic(syncopal) and epileptic mechanisms differentiated by oculocardiac reflex. Br Med J 2: 726–8.
11. Sreeram N, Whitehouse W. (1996) Permanent cardiac pacing for reflex anoxic seizure. Arch Dis Childhood75: 462.
12. McLeod KA, Wilson N, Hewitt J, et al. (1999) Cardiac pacing for severe childhood neurally mediated syncope with reflex anoxic seizures. Heart 82: 721–5.

13. Stephenson JBP, McLeod KA. (2000) Reflex anoxic seizures. In: David TJ. Recent advances in paediatrics 18. Edinburgh: Churchill Livingstone.
14. Fitzpatrick A, Sutton R. (1989) Tilting towards a diagnosis in recurrent unexplained syncope. Lancet 1:658–60.
15. Lempert T, Bauer M, Schmidt D. (1994) Syncope: A videometric analysis of 56 episodes of transient cerebral hypoxia. Ann Neurol 36: 233–7.
16. Lempert T. (1996) Recognizing syncope: Pitfalls and surprise. J Royal Soc Med 89: 372–5.
17. Camfield PR, Camfield CS. (1990) Syncope in childhood: A case control clinical study of the familial tendency to faint. Can J Neurol Sci 17: 306–8.
18. North KN, Ouvrier RA, Nugent M. (1990) Pseudoseizures caused by hyperventilation resembling absence epilepsy. J Child Neurol 5: 288–94.
19. Mathias CJ, Bannister R, Cortelli P, et al. (1990) Clinical, autonomic and therapeutic observations in two siblings with postural hypotension and sympathetic failure due to an inability to synthesize noradrenaline from dopamine because of a deficiency of dopamine betahydroxylase. Q J Med 75: 617–33.
20. Oslizlok P, Allen M, Griffin M, et al. (1992) Clinical features and management of young patients with cardioinhibitory response during orthostatic testing. Am J Cardiol 69: 1363–5.
21. Stewart JM. (2002) Orthostatic intolerance in pediatrics. J Pediatr 140: 404–11.
22. Stewart JM, Gewittz MH, Weldon A, et al. (1999) Patterns of orthostatic intolerance: The orthostatic tachycardia syndrome and adolescent chronic fatigue. J Pediatr 135: 218–25.
23. Jervell A, Lange-Nielsen F. (1957) Congenital deaf-mutism, functional heart disease with prolongation of the Q-T interval and sudden death. Am Heart J 54: 59–67.
24. Newton-Cheh C, Shah R. (2007) Genetic determinants of QT interval variation and sudden cardiac death. Curr Opin Genet Dev. 17: 1–9.
25. Culpepper N. (1737) A directory for midwives; or a guide for women in their conception, bearing (etc.). London: Bettersworth & Hitch.
26. Gordon N. (1987) Breath-holding spells. Dev Med Child Neurol 29: 810–4.
27. Breningstall GN. (1996) Breath holding spells. Pediatr Neurol 14: 91–7.
28. Dimario FJ, Burleson JA. (1993) Behaviour profile of children with severe breath-holding spells. J Pediatr 122: 488–91.
29. Southall DP, Johnson P, Morley CJ, et al. (1985) Prolonged expiratory apnoea: A disorder resulting in episodes of severe arterial hypoxaemia in infants and young children. Lancet 2:571–7.
30. Daoud S, Batieha A, al-Sheyyab M, et al. (1997) Effectiveness of iron therapy on breath holding spells. J Pediatr 130: 547–50.
31. Glaze DG, Schultz RJ, Frost JD. (1998) Rett syndrome: Characterization of seizures versus non-seizures. Electroencephal Clin Neurophysiol 106: 79–83.
32. Gastaut H, Broughton R, de Leo G. (1982) Syncopal attacks compulsively self-induced by the Valsalva manoeuvre in children with mental retardation. Electroencephal Clin Neurophysiol 35(Suppl.); 323–9.
33. Genton P, Dusserre A. (1993) Pseudo-absences atoniques par syncopes auto-provoquees (manoeuvre de Valsalva). Epilepsies 5: 223–7.
34. Horrocks IA, Nechay A, Stephenson JBP, et al. (2005) Anoxic-epileptic seizures: Observational study of epileptic seizures induced by syncopes. Arch Dis Childhood. 90: 1283–7.
35. Nechay A, Ross LM, Stephenson JBP, et al. (2004) Grastification disorder ("infantile masturbation"): A review. Arch Dis Childhood 89: 225–6.
36. Carcani-Rathwell I, Rabe- Hasketh S, Santosh PJ. (2006) Repetitive and stereotyped behaviours in pervasive developmental disorders. J Child Psych Psychiatr 47: 573–81.
37. Blackmore S. (1998) Experiences of anoxia: Do reflex anoxic seizures resemble NDEs? J Near Death Studies 17: 111–20.
38. Mahowald MW, Schenck CH. (1992) Dissociated states of wakefulness and sleep. Neurology 42(suppl.6): 44–52.
39. Ollendick TH, Mattis, SG, King NJ. (1994) Panic in children and adolescents: A review. J Child Psychol Psychiatr 35: 113–34.

40. Laidlaw JDD, Zaw KM. (1993) Epilepsy mistaken for panic attacks in an adolescent girl. Br Med J 306: 709–10.
41. Scalise A, Placidi F, Diomedi M, et al. (2006) Panic disorder or epilepsy? A case report. J Neurol Sci 246: 173–5.
42. Goodwin DS, Simms M, Bergman R. (1979) Hysterical seizures: A sequel to incest. Am J Orthopsychiatr 49: 698–703.
43. Alper K, Devinski, O, Perrine K, et al. (1993) Non epileptic seizures and childhood sexual and physical abuse. Neurology 43: 1950–3.
44. Linzer M, Varia I, Pontinen M, et al. (1992) Medically unexplained syncope: Relationship to psychiatric illness. Am J Med. 92(suppl. 1A): 18S–25S.
45. Taylor DC. (1979) The components of sickness: Diseases, illnesses, and predicaments. Lancet 2: 1008–10.
46. Gudmundsson O, Prendergast M, Foreman D, et al. (2001) Outcome of pseudoseizures in children and adolescents: A 6-year symptom survival analysis. Dev Med Child Neurol 43: 547–51.
47. Jureidini J, Taylor DC. (2002) Hysteria. Pretending to be sick. Eur Child Adoles Psy 11: 123–8.
48. Derry CP, Davey M, Johns M, et al. (2006) Distinguishing sleep disorders from seizures: Diagnosing bumps in the night. Arch Neurol 63:705–9.
49. Mason TB, Pack AI. (2005) Sleep terrors in childhood. J Pediatr 147:388–92.
50. Dalla Bernardina B, Colamaria V, Chiamenti C, et al. (1992) Benign partial epilepsy with affective symptoms (benign psychomotor epilepsy). In Roger J, Bureau M, Dravet C, Dreifuss FE, Perret A, Wolf P (eds.) Epileptic syndromes in infancy, childhood and adolescence, 2nd ed. London: John Libbey, 219–23.
51. Hickey MG, Demaarschalk BM, Caselli RJ, et al. (2007) "Idiopathic" rapid-eye-movement (REM) sleep behaviour disorder is associated with future development of neurodegenerative diseases. Neurologist 13:98–101.
52. Anderson KN, Smith IE, Schneerson JM. (2006) Rhythmic movement disorder (head banging) in an adult during rapid eye movement sleep. Movement Disord 21:866–7.
53. Fusco L, Pachatz C, Cusmai R, et al. (1999) Repetitive sleep starts in neurologically impaired children: An unusual non-epileptic manifestation in otherwise epileptic subjects. Epileptic Disord 1:63–7.
54. Challamel MJ, Mazzola ME, Nevsmalova S, et al. (1994) Narcolepsy in children. Sleep 17 (8 Suppl): S17–20.
55. Macleod S, Ferrie C, Zuberi SM. (2005) Symptoms of narcolepsy in children misinterpreted as epilepsy. Epileptic Disord 7:13–17.
56. Guilleminault C, Pelayo R. (2000) Narcolepsy in children: A practical guide to its diagnosis, treatment and follow-up. Paediatr Drugs 2:1–9.
57. Guerrini R, Aicardi J, Andermann F, Hallett M (eds.). (2002) Epilepsy and movement disorders. Cambridge, UK: Cambridge University Press.
58. Fahn S. (1994) The paroxysmal dyskinesias. In Marsden CD, Fahn S (eds.). Movement disorders 3. Oxford: Butterworth Heineman, 310–45.
59. Houser MK, Soland VL, Bhatia KP, Quinn MP, Marsden CD. (1999) Paroxysmal kinesigenic choreoathetosis: A report of 26 cases. J Neurol 246:120–6.
60. Bhatia KP, Soland VL, Bhatt MH, et al. (1997) Paroxysmal exercise induced dystonia: Eight new sporadic cases and a review of the literature. Movement Dis 12: 1007–12.
61. Browne DL, Gancher ST, Nutt JG, et al. (1994) Episodic ataxia/myokymia syndrome is associated with point mutations in the human potassium channel gene KCNA1. Nature Genet 8: 136–40.
62. Zuberi SM, Eunson LH, Spauschus A, et al. (1999) A novel mutation in the human voltage gated potassium channel gene (Kv1.1) associates with episodic ataxia and sometimes with partial epilepsy. Brain 122: 817–25.
63. Eunson LH, Rea R, Zuberi SM, et al. (2000) Clinical, genetic, and expression studies of mutations in the human voltage-gated potassium channel KCNA1 reveal new phenotypic variability. Ann Neurol 48: 647–56.

64. Gibbs J, Appleton RE. (1992) False diagnosis of epilepsy in children. Seizure 1: 15–18.
65. Thomsen LL, Eriksen MK, Roemer SF et al (2002) A population-based study of familial hemiplegic migraine suggests revised diagnostic criteria. Brain 125: 1389–91.
66. Twaijri WA, Shevell MI. (2002) Pediatric migraine equivalents: Occurrence and clinical features in practice. Pediatr Neurol 26: 365–8.
67. Verret S, Steele JC. (1971) Alternating hemiplegia in childhood: A report of eight patients with complicated migraine beginning in infancy. Pediatrics 47: 675–80.
68. Mikati MA, Kramer U, Zupanc ML, et al. (2000) Alternating hemiplegia of childhood: Xlinical manifestations and long-term outcome. Pediatr Neurol 23: 134–41.
69. Bursztyn J, Mikaeloff Y, Kaminska A, et al. (2000) Hemiplegies alternantes de l'enfant et leurs anomalies oculo-motrices [Alternating hemiplegia of childhood and oculomotor anomalies] J Fran Ophtalmol 23: 161–4.
70. Tobias ES, Tolmie JL, Stephenson JBP. (2002) Cataplexy in the Prader-Willi syndrome. Arch Dis Childhood 87: 170.
71. Crow YJ, Zuberi SM, McWilliam R, et al. (1998) "Cataplexy" and muscle ultrasound abnormalities in Coffin-Lowry syndrome. J Med Genet 35: 94–8.
72. Stephenson JBP, Hoffman MC, Russel AJ, et al. (2005) The movement disorders of Coffin-Lowry Syndrome. Brain Dev 27: 108–13.
73. Wang D, Pascual JM, Yang H, et al. (2005) Glut-1-deficiency syndrome: Clinical, genetic and therapeutic aspects. Ann Neurol 57: 111–8.

Section II
Treatment Issues

Chapter 6
Management of Acute Seizures in Persons with Intellectual Disabilities

F. M. C. Besag

Introduction

The acute management of seizures in people with intellectual disabilities (ID) comprises at least seven different situations: the first seizure, subsequent seizures/seizure exacerbations in established epilepsy, loss of skills related to frequent daytime seizures, nonconvulsive status epilepticus, loss of skills related to nocturnal seizures, electrical status epilepticus of slow wave sleep, and treatment of (convulsive) status epilepticus. These situations will be discussed in turn. Because epilepsy is not only more common in people with ID but also more difficult to treat, the emergency treatment of epilepsy is of particular importance in this group.[1] Furthermore, people with ID are sometimes prescribed other medications that may lower the seizure threshold, increasing the risk of seizures and the need for training in their acute management. Loss of skills as a result of the epilepsy is a serious matter in any patient group but can be avoided or prevented in many cases. In people with limited intellectual ability, additional loss of skills can be of major importance, emphasizing the need for a good understanding of the principles of effective epilepsy management.

The First Seizure

If the seizure is prolonged, results in injury, or is not followed by prompt return to consciousness, urgent medical attention is advisable (see below). In other cases, unless the patient is unwell or appears to have another medical condition, it will not usually be necessary to summon urgent medical attention, but it is good practice to have the patient assessed by a doctor the same day. This is particularly the case for children because many rare metabolic conditions result in seizures,[2] and the seizure may, in some cases, be the presenting feature. When the patient is seen soon after the first seizure, the specific questions that need to be answered are as follows.

Is there any identifiable precipitant?

Are investigations indicated?

Is the patient well enough to be discharged or does he/she need to be observed in hospital?

V.P. Prasher, M.P. Kerr (eds.) *Epilepsy and Intellectual Disabilities*,
DOI: 10.1007/978-1-84800-259-3_6, © Springer Science+Business Media, LLC 2008

Table 6.1 Possible causes of epilepsy include the following
(Simplified and adapted from Hopkins[2])

Idiopathic/genetic
Congenital abnormalities
Antenatal or perinatal injury
Prolonged febrile convulsions
Trauma
Infection
Cerebrovascular
Cerebral tumor
Neurodegenerative conditions
Toxins
Metabolic disorders

What plan of action should be taken if he/she has another seizure?

With regard to the cause of the seizure, the usual checklist would apply (see Table 6.1),[2] but particular attention should be drawn to the possibility of unsuspected traumatic head injury in people with motor problems as well as ID and to metabolic disorders which, as already stated, although rare, are much more likely to occur in people with ID. Meningitis and encephalitis are important acute causes of seizures and require specific medical treatment. Chin and colleagues[3] have emphasized the importance of acute bacterial meningitis as a cause of prolonged seizures in children with a fever. Other medical conditions are associated with an increased risk of seizures and may require urgent treatment; for example, hypoglycemia from an excessive insulin dose in diabetes may present as an acute seizure in people with or without epilepsy.

The decision about whether the patient is well enough to be discharged from hospital is a clinical one that will depend on such factors as the duration of the seizure (prolonged seizures lasting 20 minutes or more will be discussed in a later section), how well the patient has recovered, other medical conditions, and whether there is any actual or suspected injury. In practice, social factors may also affect the decision on the timing of discharge, for example, if the patient will be returning to capable, reliable caregivers who can cope with the situation.

The plan of action if the person has another seizure will depend greatly on some of the factors already discussed, but it would be usual for the individual to be admitted to hospital if more than one seizure occurred within 24 hours in someone who had not previously had seizures.

Subsequent Seizures/Seizure Exacerbations in Established Epilepsy

The ideal situation would be for every member of the public to know how to manage a person having a seizure. However, because this is not the case, it is necessary to provide parents and caregivers with instructions once the diagnosis of epilepsy has been made. The instructions are straightforward, but because of the mythology surrounding epilepsy, it is necessary to provide them clearly. Above all, common sense should prevail. If the person in the seizure is at risk of injury, for example, if the head is bumping against a hard surface, then the head should be held in the hands of the caregiver or should be protected in some other way, for example, by placing a soft object beneath it. A rolled-up jumper or coat can serve this purpose. Other obvious safety precautions should be taken. For example, if someone is having a seizure in the road they need to be moved to a safer place. Objects should not be put into the mouth. This may result in the patient's teeth being broken or the caregiver's fingers being bitten. Contrary to traditional false information, it is not possible for a person to swallow his or her tongue during a seizure, but the tongue may fall back into the airway at the end of the seizure, causing obstruction and, for this reason, it is advisable to place the person in the recovery position after the seizure. Confusion sometimes arises because of the instruction to put the person in the recovery position. Of course this is impossible <u>during</u> a tonic-clonic seizure, but it is an important and worthwhile measure to take <u>after</u> the seizure, to encourage a clear airway and to allow any secretions to drain.

Apart from the first seizure (see previous section) medical attention should not be required in someone who is otherwise well, with the exception of two situations: a prolonged seizure/failure to recover adequately within a few minutes of a seizure or injury in the seizure. As already discussed, if the seizure is precipitated by an underlying illness, then medical attention may also be required. It is not necessary to call an ambulance or arrange for admission to hospital if the individual recovers promptly from the seizure and is conscious but simply tired. Brief postictal confusion is common. Sometimes this confusion may lead to "resistive violence"[4]: if the person is left to recover without being approached/touched, then this is unlikely to occur but if some people are approached closely or touched soon after a seizure, while still in a confused state, they may misinterpret these actions and the caregiver may be pushed away or struck. If postictal confusion is prolonged or particularly troublesome, medical attention might be required. Some individuals are liable to postictal psychosis.[5] This may occur after "a lucid interval" of several hours or a few days.[6] Postictal psychosis is usually brief, typically lasting about one to five days, and is self-limiting, but if it is severe or associated with risk, treatment with neuroleptic medication may be indicated.

It is important for the caregivers to have an understanding of the different types of seizure that can occur. They should be provided with written information and given the opportunity to discuss this with a doctor or a specialist nurse. This also assists in seizure recording by the caregiver, which can be invaluable in the overall, longer-term management of the patient.

If a seizure exacerbation occurs in established epilepsy, then it is again necessary to try to discover whether there is an identifiable precipitant such as an intercurrent illness, failure to take the medication, or disturbed sleep pattern. Other precipitants may be responsible in particular individuals. Sometimes the pattern of the epilepsy involves having clusters of seizures, when several seizures occur over one day or over a few days. If the individual is known to have clusters of seizures, the prescription of an oral benzodiazepine such as clobazam after the second seizure of the cluster can be helpful. If the person always has clusters of seizures, then the oral benzodiazepine may be given after the first seizure (of the anticipated cluster). If giving a single dose is not effective, it may be worth considering giving the oral benzodiazepine over the expected period of the cluster. This reduces the number of seizures in at least some people. In others it appears only to delay the cluster.

In this context it is worth mentioning that some females have seizure exacerbations around the time of their menstrual period.[7,8] If this pattern is well established, giving an oral benzodiazepine such as clobazam for a few days at the right time in the menstrual cycle may greatly decrease the number of seizures or may even eliminate them altogether.

Loss of Skills Related to Frequent Daytime Seizures

I have discussed this important issue in detail elsewhere[9,10] and, because of this, will not present it in detail here. Briefly, the concept is that a person having frequent seizures may not have time to recover from one seizure before having another. They are in a constant postictal state. This can present as additional ID, which may be misinterpreted as being a permanent state, leading to misjudgments about the individual's actual ability. When the seizures are better controlled, the person emerges from the constant postictal state and functions at a much higher level. This is one of the situations of "state-dependent learning disability," which I have discussed elsewhere.[10] Although this situation might appear obvious, in practice it is easily missed, and very inappropriate decisions may be made about the ability of the individual and consequently about the facilities required for their longer-term care. It could be argued that this is not within the remit of "acute seizure management," but it is certainly in the category of urgent seizure management because the quality of life of the individual can be affected profoundly by the additional disability.

Nonconvulsive Status Epilepticus

This condition can present at any age, and it is of particular interest to note that it may do so *de novo* in the elderly, in some cases with no previous history of epilepsy.[11] The individual presents with loss of skills, of unexplained origin. Again, this has been discussed in detail elsewhere.[10,12] It is certainly a situation that requires urgent assessment and treatment. The clinical presentation of this condition is tremendously variable and, in particular, the degree of additional impairment can vary greatly from one person to another. Some are profoundly impaired during bouts of nonconvulsive status epilepticus, whereas in others the changes can be quite subtle; the individual may simply seem less capable on some occasions. Nonconvulsive status epilepticus can last for period of hours, days, or longer.

Unless the clinician thinks of the diagnosis, nonconvulsive status epilepticus may go unsuspected, undiagnosed, and untreated. In generalized nonconvulsive status epilepticus, an EEG during one of the phases of loss of ability should give an immediate diagnosis. Complex partial seizure nonconvulsive status epilepticus can be more difficult to diagnose. A detailed discussion of these conditions is beyond the remit of this chapter. However, it is worth noting that if nonconvulsive status epilepticus does not resolve rapidly it may be worth treating it with intravenous benzodiazepines, such as diazemuls. If the attacks are recurrent, then altering the regular antiepileptic medication can be beneficial. Drugs such as sodium valproate and/or lamotrigine are often highly effective.

Loss of Skills Related to Nocturnal Seizures

In a consecutive series of 24-hour video/EEG recordings of children and teenagers with epilepsy under my care, most of whom had ID, analysis of the videotapes revealed that a surprising number of these individuals were having frequent nocturnal seizures that were unobserved and unsuspected by awake night staff. Two of the boys in this series had over 200 seizures in a single night. Frequent nocturnal seizures are likely to affect daytime behavior, not only because of postictal effects but also because the seizures disrupt sleep. In some of these videotaped subjects, arousals occurred after many or most of the seizures. The seizure type that is perhaps most often missed is the brief tonic seizure. These were very evident on the split-screen video EEG records but would not have been at all obvious from the videotapes if the simultaneous EEG recordings had not been viewed. Other types of seizures may occur frequently overnight and can apparently be associated with impairment of daytime ability. A 9-year-old boy under my care had screaming episodes overnight. Videotapes (without EEG) were scrutinized by experts in sleep and epilepsy, but no diagnosis was made. Re-examination of the tapes indicated that these episodes were consistent with frontal lobe seizures. Carbamazepine had been poorly tolerated in this child, but good control was achieved with levetiracetam. His social interaction and speech development improved markedly when the seizures were controlled.

Electrical Status Epilepticus of Slow Wave Sleep

Continuous spike-wave discharges in slow wave sleep (CSWS)[13] or electrical status epilepticus of slow wave sleep (ESES) is an even more subtle form of overnight epileptic abnormality. ESES is usually defined as at least 85% of slow wave sleep being occupied by spike-wave discharges. However, it is likely that frequent epileptiform discharges not meeting the criteria for ESES are also associated with loss of skills. The classic situation of cognitive impairment in association with ESES is the Landau-Kleffner syndrome of acquired epileptic aphasia.[14,15] However, other cognitive skills, not necessarily language, may be impaired by ESES. A male patient under my care had good language skills but grossly impaired visuospatial skills. He had lost skills. He had a right porencephalic cyst. Careful assessment by the neurosurgeon revealed no obvious neurosurgical cause, such as raised intracranial pressure, for the loss of skills. Overnight EEG monitoring revealed ESES. He subsequently underwent a right hemispherectomy and the ESES resolved, with a remarkable return of his visuospatial skills.

Again, although these situations might not be viewed as requiring acute epilepsy management, they are, nevertheless, situations requiring prompt treatment, without which permanent loss of skills may, in at least some cases, occur. Robinson and colleagues[16] showed that none of the children with Landau-Kleffner syndrome who had ESES for more than 36 months subsequently had normal speech.

Treatment of (Convulsive) Status Epilepticus

Convulsive status epilepticus may be defined as a tonic-clonic (or clonic) seizure lasting longer than 20 minutes or repeated tonic-clonic (or clonic) seizures without recovery of consciousness. The term convulsive status epilepticus has now become quite widely adopted. However, I am of the opinion that this terminology has serious shortcomings because it is too narrow. If a patient continues to convulse for 20 minutes or longer, this is clearly a medical emergency, but if a patient is unconscious as a result of seizure activity of any type, for 20 minutes or longer, this constitutes a medical emergency. Rarely, tonic status epilepticus may occur with no clonic phase. I have seen this in one of my patients; the condition failed to respond to intravenous benzodiazepines, but it eventually responded to intravenous clormethiazole with a rapid return to consciousness. Some patients also seem to have prolonged atonic states in association with seizures. Whether these are ictal or postictal states may be difficult to determine from the history alone. These patients certainly need urgent medical assessment and may require urgent medical treatment.

The best approach is probably the simplest one. If any patient is unconscious for a prolonged period, this should be viewed as a medical emergency. If the unconsciousness is considered to be a direct result of the epilepsy and not, for example, the result of a head injury sustained in a seizure or another medical condition, then emergency antiepileptic treatment should be given. The other types of status epilepticus, such as complex partial seizure status epilepticus or simple partial seizure status epilepticus, in which the individual is not unconscious, certainly warrant treatment, but the situation is less urgent. There are reports of focal brain damage being associated with, and probably resulting from, prolonged focal seizure activity, but the duration of this activity has usually been days rather than minutes or hours.[17,18] In the remainder of this section the term *status epilepticus* will only be used to denote the situations in which the patient remains unconscious as a direct result of the seizure activity.

The treatment of status epilepticus has been the subject of a number of reviews and, notably, an important book.[19] Status epilepticus appears to be more likely in people with ID.[1] Although there is debate about how frequently status epilepticus causes permanent brain damage,[20] it certainly does so in some cases. Because of this, the view of many clinicians is that it should always be treated promptly so as not to put the patient at risk of permanent brain damage. There is some evidence to suggest that the more promptly status epilepticus is treated, the more likely it is to respond successfully to treatment.[21,22] This implies that a judgment needs to be made about when the patient has continued in a seizure for long enough for emergency treatment to be warranted. The usual criterion is that if the individual remains in a seizure for five minutes or longer then urgent treatment should be given. However, the care plan should be tailored to the seizure history. For example, if a patient is known always to go into status epilepticus if the seizure lasts longer than one or two minutes, then the emergency treatment might be given at that stage. If, on the other hand, a patient who is known to go into status epilepticus, frequently has seizures lasting six minutes, which then usually resolve without treatment, as was the case for one of my patients, a different care plan would be indicated. In this case it would be appropriate to wait for six minutes before administering the emergency treatment, so as to avoid unnecessary treatment, but then to intervene promptly if the seizure were continuing.

Because transfer to hospital is typically likely to take at least 20 minutes, pre-hospital treatment is usually appropriate. For individuals who are known to go into status epilepticus, the parents/caregivers should be trained in the emergency treatment of this condition. The treatments that can be administered by nonmedical personnel include rectal diazepam, rectal paraldehyde, intranasal midazolam, or buccal midazolam. These treatments will be discussed in turn.

Generally it is good practice to arrange for the patient to be seen by a doctor or to be taken to an emergency department of a hospital if out-of-hospital treatment for status epilepticus has been required. However, there are exceptions. If the caregivers are experienced, confident, and competent, having previously managed this situation for the patient, the need to involve a doctor may be left to their discretion. These general comments apply regardless of the type of out-of-hospital emergency treatment given, whether it is rectal diazepam or one of the other options discussed in this section. Out-of-hospital treatment should only be administered by individuals who have been properly trained and should only be administered to patients according to a clear, individualized emergency care plan, with consent/agreement from the patient, parent, or other person/agency responsible for the patient. For example, if the child is in the care of the social services department, the written approval of that department would be required. If the person administering the emergency treatment is a member of staff and not the parent, then there is a strong argument for insisting that they not only have the necessary training but that they are also certified as being approved to administer the treatment by their employer. No nonmedical personnel should be expected to administer emergency medication unless they are willing to do so, properly trained, competent and confident with regard to both the procedure and the situation.

Rectal Diazepam

This is a well-established and effective treatment in most cases.[23] Although it is used worldwide, it is interesting to note that a rectal preparation for diazepam (diastat rectal gel)[24] has only been available in the United States for relatively few years. The usual dose is up to 0.5mg/kg in a child or up to 30mg in an adult. In practice, if the individual weighs over 20kg, 10mg is given in the first instance. If the seizure is not clearly abating (or if consciousness is not being regained) approximately five minutes after the rectal diazepam has been administered, then further doses may be given up to the maximum of 0.5mg/kg. As a general rule, if the first dose is not effective, arrangements should be made for urgent transfer to hospital.

Rectal Paraldehyde

This may be prescribed if the patient is known to be resistant to benzodiazepines or has a history of adverse effects to benzodiazepines. It is also sometimes prescribed as a second-line treatment if a benzodiazepine has failed. The usual convention is to mix the paraldehyde with an equal volume of oil on the basis that this might reduce the possibility of rectal ulceration, but there seems to be no clearly documented good evidence that this is necessary and it complicates treatment. Mixing with oil delays treatment and might also delay absorption of the paraldehyde. I have always administered the paraldehyde without oil. It can be flushed through with tap water. In the past, glass syringes were used because of concern that the paraldehyde might dissolve plastic syringes. With the plastic syringes currently in use, this does not appear to be a problem, but it is usual practice to give the paraldehyde promptly and not to leave it for long periods in the syringe. Paraldehyde appears to be safe, provided it has not decomposed, when it can be potentially toxic. The vial should always be inspected. The fluid should resemble clear water. If it is discolored it should be discarded. Paraldehyde has a strong odor. Some people find this unpleasant. Because it is excreted through the lungs, the patient's breath will smell of paraldehyde for some time after it has been administered.

It would be possible, at least in theory, for intramuscular paraldehyde to be given as prehospital treatment, but this would not be recommended because of potential adverse effects; in particular, sterile abscesses have been reported at the injection site and if the injection is incorrectly placed, damage to the sciatic nerve might occur.

Nasal (Intranasal) Midazolam

Reports of successful treatment of status epilepticus with intranasal midazolam[25–28] appeared at about the same time as those on buccal midazolam (see next section). Because of the proximity of the upper cavity with the nose and the brain, the nasal route might offer particular advantages for rapid brain penetration. The proportion of liquid midazolam squirted into the nose that reaches the cerebral circulation in this way remains uncertain. In practice, nasal midazolam is effective as prehospital treatment of status epilepticus. It has obvious advantages over rectal diazepam. It has been suggested that there may also be disadvantages of this route. As the patient breathes, some of the liquid might be discharged out of the nose. If there are copious nasal secretions, this may make reliable administration more difficult. In a patient who is jerking violently, aiming to insert something into the nostril to administer the midazolam could be difficult or even hazardous. There has been some debate about whether this route or the buccal route (see next section) is to be preferred.[29,30]

Buccal Midazolam

I recall having heard a colleague speak of treating status epilepticus by placing clonazepam into the mouth and allowing it to be absorbed through the oral mucosa if intravenous access was difficult. However, there was no published work on the use of the buccal route of benzodiazepine administration for status epilepticus or for any other indication. Because of this, I suggested to an associate of the appropriate pharmaceutical firm that a study might be performed to determine if buccal/sublingual diazepam could be used instead of rectal diazepam as out-of-hospital treatment for status epilepticus. This discussion was carried out in the presence of Professor Brian Neville, who supported the idea and became involved in the research from the outset. The pharmaceutical company recommended buccal midazolam rather than buccal diazepam. The research was successfully completed by Dr. Rod Scott and published.[31,32] Since then, this method of treatment has been very widely used. A more recent randomized study (in which I was not involved) compared children who were given rectal diazepam with those who received buccal midazolam in the emergency room.[33] The authors concluded that, dose for dose, buccal midazolam was superior to rectal diazepam and was not associated with more adverse effects. The results of this study were convincing in terms of efficacy, but it should be pointed out that it was not sufficiently powered to draw firm conclusions regarding differences in relatively infrequent adverse effects, such as serious respiratory depression. Although there have been no major concerns about the safety of buccal midazolam, more data are required before a definitive statement on safety can be made. What does not remain in doubt is the combination of efficacy and convenience of this treatment. These comments are perhaps particularly true for some patients with ID, especially those with mobility problems. Trying to administer rectal diazepam in a large person having a tonic-clonic seizure in a wheelchair, for example, could prove to be very difficult, whereas administering buccal midazolam is straightforward. Nasal midazolam could, of course, also be administered in this situation, but placing liquid into the mouth is probably much easier than placing it into the nose. It does not seem to matter if the patient swallows some of the fluid; the action appears to be just as rapid. There are many other situations in which administering buccal midazolam would be more convenient and less embarrassing than administering rectal diazepam. For example, administering rectal diazepam in a crowded underground railway carriage might be problematic. In addition there have been growing concerns about the personal privacy of patients and about the possibility of staff being accused of impropriety when it is necessary to remove the lower clothing to administer rectal diazepam.

Buccal midazolam is not licensed for any indication. In the UK, midazolam is not licensed, via any route, for the treatment of status epilepticus, although it has been shown to be effective.[32, 34] Despite this and despite the lack of extensive safety data, the convenience and efficacy of this treatment appear to have been influential, resulting in its widespread use.

Emergency Treatment of Status Epilepticus in Hospital

The principles underlying the in-hospital treatment of status epilepticus in people with or without ID are no different. However, as already discussed, status epilepticus appears to be more common and more difficult to treat in people with ID. It is worth repeating the point that has already been made about the importance of treating promptly, not only because it decreases the probability of brain damage but also because the status epilepticus seems to be much more responsive to treatment if the latter is given early. Prompt treatment can avoid the more difficult-to-treat established status epilepticus. If prompt out-of-hospital treatment is given by the parent or caregiver, hospital treatment may be avoided altogether. However, if treatment in the emergency room, general ward, or intensive care unit is required, there are well-established protocols that can be followed.[19,35–37] These generally recommend that if treatment with full doses of a benzodiazepine such as diazepam, lorazepam, clonazepam, or midazolam via the rectal/buccal or parenteral route have not been effective, then a phenytoin/fosphenytoin infusion should be commenced, typically in a dose of 18mg/kg phenytoin or equivalent. If this fails to control the status epilepticus a barbiturate and/or anesthetic agent may be used. However, while working in an epilepsy center with an emergency room but no on-site intensive care facilities, I have found that other strategies can be useful. As already stated, rectal paraldehyde can be effective when benzodiazepines have failed. Another option is intravenous chlormethiazole, which can be very effective when other drugs have not controlled the status epilepticus. There have been concerns about the possibility of life-threatening respiratory depression with this drug, but if it is injected slowly by the doctor, rather than being left as an intravenous drip (with the potential of excessive doses being given unsupervised), it is, in my experience, both safe and valuable.

Conclusion

People with ID have a greater probability of developing epilepsy, are more likely to have seizures that are resistant to treatment, and are at greater risk of status epilepticus, which can cause further impairment and is associated with a high mortality rate. In addition to convulsive status epilepticus, there are several situations in which the epilepsy may cause worsening of the ID. Prompt recognition and effective treatment can, in many cases, prevent this additional morbidity and mortality. A high degree of awareness in caregivers and professionals is an essential first step in preventing these problems. This, in turn, depends on high standards of education and training, which should be mandatory in those responsible for the management of people with ID and epilepsy.

References

1. Pellock JM, Morton LD. (2000) Treatment of epilepsy in the multiply handicapped. Ment Retard Dev D R 6:309-323.
2. Hopkins A. (1995) The causes of epilepsy, the risk factors for epilepsy and the precipitation of seizures. In: Hopkins A, Shorvon S, Cascino GD (eds). Epilepsy. London: Chapman & Hall Medical. 59–85.
3. Chin RF, Neville BG, Scott RC, et al. (2005) Meningitis is a common cause of convulsive status epilepticus with fever. Arch Dis Childhood 90:66–69.
4. Treiman DM. (1991) Psychobiology of ictal aggression. Advan Neurol 55:341–356.
5. Logsdail SJ, Toone BK. (1988) Post-ictal psychoses. A clinical and phenomenological description. Br J Psychiatr 152:246–252.
6. Kanner AM. (2000) Psychosis of epilepsy: A neurologist's perspective. Epilepsy Behav 1:219–227.
7. Crawford P. (2005) Best practice guidelines for the management of women with epilepsy. Epilepsia 46: (Suppl 9):117–124.
8. O'Brien MD, Gilmour-White SK. (2005) Management of epilepsy in women. Postgrad Med J 81:278–285.
9. Besag FMC. (2003) The EEG and learning disability. In: Trimble M (ed.). Learning disability and epilepsy — An integrative approach. Guildford: Clarius Press, 111–131.
10. Besag FMC. (2001) Treatment of state-dependent learning disability. Epilepsia 42 (Suppl. 1):52–54.
11. Sheth RD, Drazkowski JF, Sirven JI, et al. (2006) Protracted ictal confusion in elderly patients. Arch Neurol 63:529–532.
12. Besag FMC. (2002) Subtle cognitive and behavioural effects of epilepsy. In: Trimble M, Schmitz B (eds.). The neuropsychiatry of epilepsy. Cambridge University Press, Cambridge:70–80.
13. Patry G, Lyagoubi S, Tassinari CA. (1971) Subclinical "electrical status epilepticus" induced by sleep in children. A clinical and electroencephalographic study of six cases. Arch Neurol 24: 242–252.
14. Landau WM, Kleffner FR. (1957) Syndrome of acquired aphasia with convulsive disorder in children. Neurology (Minneap) 7: 523–530.
15. Tassinari CA, Rubboli G, Volpi L, . et al. (2000) Encephalopathy with electrical status epilepticus during slow sleep or ESES syndrome including the acquired aphasia. Clin Neurophysiol 111(Suppl 2): S94–S102.

16. Robinson RO, Baird G, Robinson G, et al. (2001) Landau-Kleffner syndrome: Course and correlates with outcome. Dev Med Child Neurol 43:243–247.
17. Donaire A, Carreno M, Gomez B, et al. (2006) Cortical laminar necrosis related to prolonged focal status epilepticus. J Neurol, Neurosurg Psychiatr 77:104–106.
18. Hilkens PH, de Weerd AW. (1995) Non-convulsive status epilepticus as cause for focal neurological deficit. Acta Neurol Scand 92:193–197.
19. Shorvon S. (1994) Status epilepticus its clinical features and treatment in children and adults. Cambridge:Cambridge University Press.
20. Shinnar S, Pellock JM, Berg AT, et al. (2001). Short-term outcomes of children with febrile status epilepticus. Epilepsia 42:47–53.
21. Pellock JM, Marmarou A, DeLorenzo R. (2004)Time to treatment in prolonged seizure episodes. Epilepsy Behav 5:192–196.
22. Kutlu NO, Dogrul M, Yakinci C, et al. (2003) Buccal midazolam for treatment of prolonged seizures in children. Brain Dev 25:275–278.
23. Franzoni E, Carboni C, Lambertini A. (1983) Rectal diazepam: A clinical and EEG study after a single dose in children. Epilepsia 24:35–41.
24. O'Del lC, Shinnar S, Ballaban-Gil KR, et al. (2005) Rectal diazepam gel in the home management of seizures in children. Pediatr Neurol 33:166–172.
25. O'Regan ME, Brown JK, Clarke M. (1996) Nasal rather than rectal benzodiazepines in the management of acute childhood seizures? Dev Med Child Neurol 38:1037–1045.
26. Scheepers M, Scheepers B, Clough P. (1998) Midazolam via the intranasal route: an effective rescue medication for severe epilepsy in adults with learning disability. Seizure 7:509–512.
27. Harbord MG, Kyrkou NE, Kyrkou MR, et al. (2004) Use of intranasal midazolam to treat acute seizures in paediatric community settings. J Paedr Child Health 40:556–558.
28. Wolfe TR, Macfarlane TC. (2006) Intranasal midazolam therapy for pediatric status epilepticus. Am J Emerg Med 24:343–346.
29. Scheepers M, Comish S, Cordes L, et al. (1999) Buccal midazolam and rectal diazepam for epilepsy. Lancet 353:1797–1798.
30. Ellis SJ, Baddely L, Scott RC, et al. (1999). Buccal midazolam and rectal diazepam for epilepsy (multiple letters) [2]. Lancet 353:1796–1798.
31. Scott RC, Besag FM, Boyd SG et al. (1998) Buccal absorption of midazolam: pharmacokinetics and EEG pharmacodynamics. Epilepsia 39:290–294.
32. Scott RC, Besag FMC, Neville BGR. (1999) Buccal midazolam and rectal diazepam for treatment of prolonged seizures in childhood and adolescence: A randomised trial. Lancet 353: 623–626.
33. McIntyre J, Robertson S, Norris E et al. (2005) Safety and efficacy of buccal midazolam versus rectal diazepam for emergency treatment of seizures in children: A randomised controlled trial. Lancet 366:205–210.
34. Pellock JM. (1998) Use of midazolam for refractory status epilepticus in pediatric patients. J Child Neurol 13:581–587.
35. Chen JW, Wasterlain CG. (2006) Status epilepticus: Pathophysiology and management in adults. Lancet Neurol 5:246–256.
36. Eriksson K, Kalviainen R. (2005) Pharmacologic management of convulsive status epilepticus in childhood. Expert Rev Neurother 5:777–783.
37. Treiman DM, Walker MC. (2006) Treatment of seizure emergencies: Convulsive and non-convulsive status epilepticus. Epilepsy Res 68(Suppl 1): S77–S82.

Chapter 7
The Use of Antiepileptic Medication in Adults with Intellectual Disabilities

J. Wilcox and M. P. Kerr

Introduction

The decision to treat epilepsy is based on an evaluation of the impact of seizures versus the potential positive and negative effects of medication. Ongoing seizures may not only have profound effects upon the physical health, cognitive state, and psychological well-being of the individual concerned, but can also have significant social consequences and costs to family life. Seizure disorders are often complex when seen in combination with intellectual disabilities (ID); the patient is more likely to experience multiple seizure types and be more refractory to treatment than those in the general population. Furthermore the common complications of physical, psychiatric, and behavioral comorbidity, along with communication impairment and multiple caregivers, add challenges to the process of prescribing and evaluating antiepileptic drug therapy.

Treatment itself may not be straightforward; there is the potential for side effects, toxicity, or pharmacological interaction with other drugs. Daily medication may serve as a constant reminder of the condition to patient and family, as well as have a stigma of its own. Relatively few randomized trials have been conducted specifically in the population of people with ID, and therefore choice of medication has to be largely based on data extrapolated from the general population and on peer experience.

Evaluating the Impact of Seizures

There may be wide individual variation in the impact of seizures upon health and social life; therefore it is important to assess this influence prior to initiating treatment or changing current treatment. People with ID and epilepsy are at greater risk of fracture, accident, and hospitalization secondary to seizures.[1] The standard mortality ratio is increased, both in those with epilepsy and the learning disabled. For those with both ID and epilepsy the figure may be as high as five times that of the general population.[2] A chronic seizure disorder may also impact upon intellectual functioning—repeated head injury can result in permanent neurological damage, or a cognitive decline may occur after prolonged status epilepticus.

V.P. Prasher, M.P. Kerr (eds.) *Epilepsy and Intellectual Disabilities*,
DOI: 10.1007/978-1-84800-259-3_7, © Springer Science+Business Media, LLC 2008

Seizures may also reduce an individual's opportunity to integrate socially and place limits upon independence. This may either be a direct result of the seizures themselves or due to beliefs held about epilepsy by family, caregivers, or society. The precise contribution of epilepsy as a source of stress when caring for someone with ID has received little attention within the literature; however, it is thought to be associated with higher levels of anxiety and depression. Surveys of the non-ID population have particularly highlighted periods of status epilepticus, severity of atonic and tonic seizures and perceived lack of support as factors which may have the greatest impact on the development of depression amongst caregivers. Other general concerns may be with regard to the fit frequency and unpredictability, specific worries around fit management and risk of injury, medication, and restrictions to the individual's lifestyle.

When to Start Treatment

The diagnosis of a seizure disorder should have been established without doubt prior to commencing treatment. This will usually be based upon a comprehensive history from a reliable witness and, where possible, the patients themselves, along with appropriate investigation, which is likely to include EEG recording and in some cases neuroimaging (see Chapter 4). A trial of anticonvulsants is unlikely to be helpful where there are uncertainties over the correct diagnosis,[3] and it is of greater benefit to seek out or await more clinical information. The diagnostic process is important in identifying seizure type and syndrome and underlying etiology of associated ID, all of which have implications for potential treatment.

Confirmation of the diagnosis of a seizure disorder does not automatically lead to pharmacological treatment as the next step. An individualized assessment of the potential impact of treatment versus the possible consequences and likelihood of a recurrence may help clarify the most appropriate time to commence treatment. In the United Kingdom (UK) it is current practice to defer treatment until two or more unprovoked seizures have occurred, the argument for this delay being that only a proportion of patients will go on to develop further seizures. A meta analysis by Berg and Shinnar in 1991[4] reported an average of 51% (range 23–71%) of those in the 17 studies they looked at went on to experience further seizures following a single initial event. Those perceived to be at higher risk of further seizures were individuals with a grossly abnormal electroencephalogam (EEG) or a structural brain lesion. It is likely that treatment halves the risk of future seizures after a first episode. It may be debated whether delaying treatment until a second seizure is seen affects prognosis or response to medication. It has been suggested that failure to achieve seizure control early on rendered an individual more resistant to treatment by causing structural brain changes and thus facilitating future events. An opposing view is that early treatment in itself has little influence on long-term outcome and that epilepsy in any individual patient has an inherent severity and response to therapy. As a consequence, more severely affected patients are more difficult to control and experience more frequent seizures from early on in their condition. The Multicentre study of Early Epilepsy and Single Seizures (1993–2002) randomized patients in whom the clinicians were unsure as to the commencement of treatment (first seizures, minor seizures, infrequent seizures) to receive either immediate therapy or to defer until treatment was clearly imperative. The authors looked at both short-term (time to first seizure) and long-term outcomes (time to two-year remission). The time to first seizure was reduced in the immediate treatment group, but by year six the number receiving drug treatment was the same in both groups (40%). The authors concluded that immediate treatment may offer some possible benefit in the first couple of years, but that it was unlikely to be of any greater clinical benefit than delayed treatment in the longer term. It is important to recognize that studies specific to people with ID do not exist.

Choosing Medication

It is estimated that between 50% and 70% of all people suffering from epilepsy will become seizure free on a single anticonvulsant. However, for a number of reasons, it is likely that this figure is significantly lower within the learning-disabled population. This relatively high incidence of resistant or difficult-to-treat seizures makes the appropriate choice of first-line therapy all the more crucial.

A detailed knowledge of both the individual patient and the potential medication is essential to make an informed decision on therapy. Ideally a medication should be effective, well tolerated during initiation, have minimal long-term side effects, and a low risk of toxicity or rare life-threatening idiopathic reactions. Of particular relevance to the ID population, consideration must be given to blood monitoring requirements and the type of preparation available.

It remains something of an aspiration that knowing the mechanism of action of a drug will help in predicting treatment outcome. Recent years have seen considerable advances in the understanding of anticonvulsant action at a cellular level. Seizure activity occurs as the result of intermittent and excessive neuronal hyperexcitablity. Anticonvulsants function by attempting to rebalance neuronal excitation and inhibition, either by modulating voltage-gated ion channels, increasing gamma—amino-butyric acid (GABA)-mediated inhibitory transmission or by attenuating glutamate-related excitation.

It is generally accepted that recognition of seizure type and syndrome will aid prediction of the most effective treatment. This is not always straightforward in people with ID; early history may be more likely to be incomplete, the patient may not be able to cooperate fully with history taking or investigation, and the probability of more than one seizure type being present is comparatively high. In the UK, carbamazepine, lamotrigine, levetiracetam, sodium valproate, and topiramate are all licensed as monotherapy for partial seizures. In the case of generalized seizures, sodium valproate and lamotrigine are generally accepted to be first-line options, though recent studies of levetiracetam in juvenile myoclonic epilepsy suggest its value in generalized seizures. Where doubt exists about type, it may be prudent to treat as if generalized seizures with a broad-spectrum drug. The difference in efficacy between treatment options is small, though as outcome is a composite of efficacy and tolerability, individual assessment of side effect potential is crucial. In a population where mental disorder and the prescription of psychotropic medication are common, consideration must also be given for potential interaction between already established medications and the proposed anticonvulsant. For example, the risk of neurotoxicity is increased with the prescription of both carbamazepine and lithium, and the potential hematological complications arising from carbamazepine and clozapine may make the combination prohibitive. Figures 7.1 and 7.2 highlight our preferred treatment algorism for mono and add-on therapy respectively.

Prescribers should also be particularly aware of their choice of AEDs when treating women with child-bearing potential. Indvidual disruption of the teratogenic risk of AEDs is beyond the remit of this chapter, but updated information should always be sought.

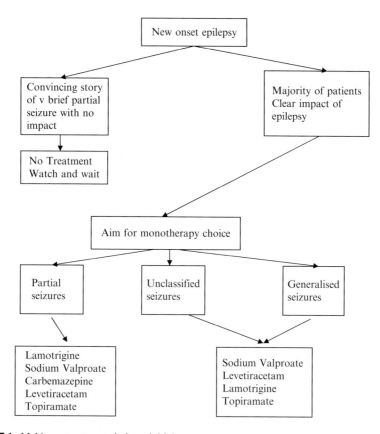

Fig. 7.1 Making a treatment choice—initial treatment

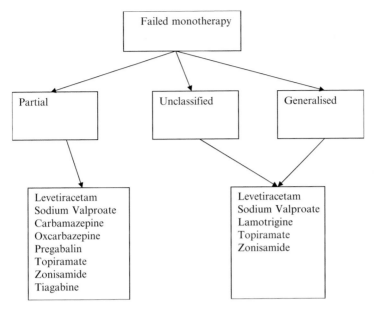

Fig. 7.2 Making a choice—monotherapy failure

Managing Medication

In most situations the advantages of a low starting dose and slow titration will out-weigh those of a more rapid introduction. The incidence of an allergic response or a dose-related side effect and consequent withdrawal from medication is less common. There is greater opportunity for identifying the minimum effective dose and less chance of missing the "therapeutic window," above which worsening of seizure control may occur, as has happened with some individuals. This approach may also be particularly beneficial in those individuals who metabolize drugs more slowly. The main disadvantage to a cautious introduction is the potential for a lengthier time to seizure control. In some cases this might result in patients or their families losing confidence in the medication, something which may be lessened by the discussion of realistic expectations of the medication prior to initiation.

There may be wide interindividual variability in rate of drug clearance, tolerance, and requirements for seizure control, which makes it difficult to estimate a target dose. For example, the rate of clearance of lamotrigine may vary by up to six times between individuals. Where seizures are frequent, the concept of a target dose is of little relevance; the dose can simply be titrated up if seizures occur. It is when seizures are rare that a target dose or blood level may be helpful, otherwise gaining seizure control may be a very lengthy process. Most patients will respond to low-to-average doses of medication; open studies often report that those who achieve seizure freedom do so with relatively small quantities.[5] Although it is common practice if complete seizure freedom has not been achieved to titrate up to the maximally tolerated dose, it is worth weighing the comparatively small potential for increased efficacy against the probability of side effects. In the patient who is still tolerating the drug but who has not gained seizure freedom, it may be worth considering splitting doses further as relatively high doses are reached.

Adverse Effects

Knowledge of the side effect profiles of the various anticonvulsants is of importance, as the learning disabled may be both particularly susceptible to developing adverse events and less able to communicate about them effectively. Adverse effects may be acute and usually dose related, idiosyncratic, or linked to chronic administration. In the general population anticonvulsants have been linked to the precipitation of delirium, psychosis, and cognitive changes. Drugs which more are more commonly known to affect cognition, such as primidone, phenytoin, or topiramate, may require careful monitoring in people with ID.

Several antiepileptic drugs (AEDs) have been found to predispose to significant change in weight. In a population where obesity is already common this should be considered before initiating treatment; valproate, gabapentin, and pregabalin are potentially associated with weight gain. Conversely, anorexia can also be problematic for a minority, and the prescription of topiramate or zonisamide may result in a loss of weight and appetite. The development of osteoporosis is associated with chronic anticonvulsant administration. This is of particular relevance to the ID population, as many will have significant co-existing risk factors for decreased bone density and fracture. Immobility, lack of exposure to sunlight, poor dietary intake of vitamin D, early menopause, and coprescription of antipsychotics are all more common amongst the ID population and may contribute to poor bone mineralization. It is unclear as to the exact mechanism by which anticonvulsants predispose to osteoporosis; possibly through the enzymatic induction of vitamin D, but decreased bone density has been reported with administration of phenytoin, phenobarbitone, primidone, carbamazepine, and valproate. Behavioral disturbance is often reported in the context of a new or increase in anticonvulsant prescription. In a population where the incidence of both epilepsy and behavioral problems is common, cause and effect is often very difficult to establish. Prior to any medication changes it is often helpful to document baseline behaviors in order that a more objective assessment may be possible following the introduction of a new drug. Should a change in behavior type or frequency then take place, there may be several possible causes other than medications. The behavior may be the consequence of improved seizure control as the patient becomes more alert and responsive. The new anticonvulsant may result in a previously rapidly generalizing partial epilepsy subsequently manifesting as an aura only, to which the patient responds fearfully. Alternatively, the possibility of adverse physical effects from the drug, such as ataxia, diplopia, or gastric irritation, should also be considered as an explanation for behavioral change.

Paradoxical Worsening of Seizures

In some instances a patient's seizure control may deteriorate on treatment. There may be a number of reasons for this. An irregular intake of medication in patients who have difficulty with the particular preparation, forget medication, or who are reluctant to comply with therapy may precipitate withdrawal seizures. Alternatively, an individual who has taken too much medication and becomes toxic may also present with seizures. Tolerance is associated with a number of anticonvulsants, in particular benzodiazepines, resulting in a progressive increase in frequency and severity of seizures. In other cases, the side effects of a drug can have direct consequences on seizure frequency. For example, increased somnolence may lead to an increase in seizure activity in a patient who experiences sleep-related seizures.

Direct aggravation by AED effect is possible. Typical absences are commonly reported to be aggravated by the use of carbamazepine, vigabatrin, tiagabine, and phenytoin. The effect of lamotrigine upon myoclonic jerks appears unpredictable in some cases; Biraben and colleagues[6] reported a deterioration in control in certain individuals. Although the clinician should recognize all these potentially drug-related causes of seizure deterioration, non-AED-related effects are important. These include natural variation in seizure frequency and altered recording by staff homes. Randomized controlled trials in individuals with ID tend to show a range of placebo-related seizure change from a decrease by 10% to an increase of 10%. It may be valuable in clinical practice to consider a variation of greater than 10% from usual being a potential AED-related effect.

Substituting and Adding Anticonvulsants

In the event the patient develops an idiosyncratic drug reaction, is unable to tolerate the first drug, or experiences a worsening of seizure control, the first medication should be substituted with a second appropriately chosen anticonvulsant. If lack of efficacy appears to be the problem, it is worth reexamining the clinical scenario before considering polytherapy—by reevaluating the original diagnosis of epilepsy, the possibility of nonepileptic seizures, the accuracy of the assessment of seizure type, compliance with medication, and the suitability of the first anticonvulsant. Consideration should also be given to the possibility of a progressive cerebral disorder.

The usual practice is to switch drugs, that is, to add in a new medication to a low treatment dose, then remove the first. Depending on the efficacy and tolerance to the second AED, a decision may then be made as to the possibility of withdrawing one of the medications. In some cases, patients who become seizure free on the combination may then develop seizures again once the first, presumed largely ineffective, AED is withdrawn. It is possible that some combinations of drugs with differing main mechanisms of action are of synergistic benefit and offer a greater degree of seizure control than could be predicted from their success as monotherapy.[7] The combination of valproate with lamotrigine is suggested to be potentially synergistic.

In the situation where the first drug is of clear benefit and well tolerated but seizure freedom has not been achieved, a second anticonvulsant may be chosen as long-term add-on therapy. When choosing a second anticonvulsant, care must be given to its potential to cause pharmacokinetic or dynamic interaction with the first. Pharmacokinetic interactions involve the alteration of a drug's concentration at the point of action by affecting absorption, distribution, metabolism, or elimination. Of particular relevance to the ID population, in whom gastric reflux is common, the prescription of antacids may affect absorption of phenytoin, carbamazepine, and gabapentin. It is also recognized that certain nasogastric feeds can significantly reduce the absorption of phenytoin. Most AEDs undergo hepatic metabolism prior to excretion. Drugs that stimulate hepatic enzymes include carbamazepine, phenytoin, phenobarbitone, and primidone, whereas sodium valproate causes inhibition. Toxic effects are a possibility where the levels of the original medication are raised by the introduction of the second AED. Many of the older drugs in particular have a narrow therapeutic range, and the plasma level that confers optimal seizure control may be very close to that which is associated with unwanted effects. Of equal concern, worsening of seizure control may occur if interaction leads to a decrease in levels of the first. Lamotrigine may be particularly problematic in this respect, since it requires differing initiation regimens when combined with a hepatic enzyme inducer or inhibitor. Anticonvulsants that do not undergo hepatic metabolism prior to excretion include levetiracetam, gabapentin, pregabalin, and vigabatrin.

Pharmacodynamic interactions occur at the cellular level when two drugs have similar mechanisms of action. For example, the combination of carbamazepine and lamotrigine, two Na-channel blockers, may be poorly tolerated because of their additive neurotoxic side effects. The GABA-ergic inhibition of both valproate and phenobarbitone may result in profound sedation, and the use of valproate with lamotrigine may present risk of significant tremor. Figure 7.2 shows an algorithm reflecting the our choices in the add-on situation.

Drug Monitoring

A clear indication for drug level monitoring is necessary if it is to be of clinical benefit. When phenytoin is prescribed, serum levels are helpful when an adjustment of dosage is considered. This drug's zero-order kinetics means that there is a narrow safety margin, and small increments in dose can lead to dramatic changes in blood concentration. There is commonly a good correlation between toxicity and serum level. For other drugs this relationship may not be so well defined; regular serum monitoring without the suspicion of toxicity can lead to unnecessary reduction of medication in individuals tolerating their current blood concentration and thus risk of loss of seizure control. Similarly, a low blood level in someone whose seizures are adequately controlled should not result in increased dosage, thus making adverse effects more likely. Other situations where drug monitoring may be of benefit include the confirmation of treatment adherence and situations when it may be predicted that a pharmacokinetic interaction will take place.

Withdrawing Medication

The 1991 MRC drug withdrawal study[8] demonstrated that ID should not necessarily be a barrier to anticonvulsant withdrawal. Forty percent of seizure-free patients were successfully able to withdraw therapy. However, because of the comparatively high incidence of refractory epilepsy among this population, many patients will require lifelong treatment. The decision to begin the slow withdrawal of medication must be based upon an evaluation of the potential benefits of anticonvulsant freedom versus risk of seizure recurrence. The potential benefits to medication withdrawal may be difficult to quantify, and assessments of individuals and their particular circumstances are required. Similarly, the potential impact of seizure recurrence may vary widely between patients and necessitate debate. It is estimated that withdrawing treatment probably doubles the risk of further seizures, with the greatest risk of recurrence in the two years post withdrawal. The risk of further seizures may vary widely, but a number of risk factors are thought to be associated with poorer outcome. Individuals suffering from severe ID and gross neurological deficits have a high probability of seizure recurrence. It is also suggested that those with a history of myoclonus or generalized tonic clonic seizures are at particularly high risk of relapse, possibly 70–80%. Those receiving polytherapy have a tendency to do worse than those whose seizures have been controlled by a single drug. In children, an abnormal EEG prior to therapy withdrawal is associated with a recurrence of seizures, but the validity of this when applied to the adult population appears uncertain. A more successful outcome may be predicted in those who have experienced a longer period of seizure freedom and fewer seizures prior to complete control and who have been found to have lower blood levels of anticonvulsant prior to reduction.

Individual Medications

A detailed knowledge of individual AEDs is essential to any clinician involved in the care of people with ID. This arguably is of equal value to family members and caregivers to help in identifying side effects in individuals. Appendix I details individual drugs and highlights potential issues of relevance within the population of people with a ID.

Specific Evidence for Antiepileptic Drugs in People with ID

It is accepted practice that wherever possible the prescription of treatment should be evidence based. In the pharmacological treatment of epilepsy this will include examining material concerning efficacy, i.e., seizure control, harmful effects, and potential drug interactions relevant to the patient in question. Different study designs are necessary to provide the range of information required. Randomized, controlled trials are often time-limited and provide information on short-term efficacy and the common early adverse events seen on initiation, but the chronic or rare side effects of a drug may not become apparent until open studies are conducted over longer periods or in special patient populations. Long-term retention studies can be useful in providing a composite measure of "therapeutic efficiency"; a drug's tolerability and efficacy may be estimated by the number of patients continuing to take it. Despite a rapid expansion in the number of randomized, controlled trials conducted on epilepsy over recent years, very few have focused on treatment in indivduals with ID. Difficulty in defining seizure type, ensuring compliance, measuring treatment outcomes, consent issues, and the high incidence of comorbidity may account for the paucity of this type of evidence. Of the few trials that have recruited from the ID population, treatment of Lennox-Gastaut syndrome has been the focus of two. The first, by Motte in 1997,[9] demonstrated the efficacy of lamotrigine and revealed relatively few side effects. The second[10] reported a reduction in seizure frequency with use of topiramate but an apparent increase in behavioral problems and a medication dropout rate of almost 30%. An alternative randomized, controlled trial conducted by Kerr in 2005[11] in an adult intellectually disabled population did not find any significant behavioral change from baseline with the prescription of topiramate, though it also showed only a trend to seizure improvement.

Most of the literature looking at anticonvulsant use in individuals with ID concerns open, noncontrolled studies or cohort studies. In a randomized open label study of gabapentin and lamotrigine in adults with ID and resistant epilepsy, Crawford and colleagues[12] reported both in both groups an approximate 50% reduction of seizures in half the patients receiving the drug. Both appeared to be equally well tolerated and associated with improvements in challenging behavior. In another open-label study focusing on people with ID and refractory epilepsy, 64 patients were prescribed adjunctive leviteracetam.[13] Thirty-eight percent were described as seizure free, a significant proportion of whom were taking just 500mg per day. A number of cohort studies have looked at the reduction of medication in this population. A 1989 study by Collacott[14] reported a reduction in the mean number of anticonvulsants taken by a cohort of 172 patients from 1.41 to 1.05 over a period of three years. The outcome appeared mixed; around half experienced a reduction in seizure frequency, one third, an increase, and the remainder were largely unchanged. Alvarez[15] also reported on the discontinuation of medication in 50 patients remaining seizure free for a minimum of two years. Over an eight-year follow-up seizures recurred in 26 patients, the majority occurring in the three-year period following reduction in medication. Predictors of successful withdrawal of medication appeared to reflect those found by other studies in the general population, as detailed in the section "Withdrawing Medication."

Evaluating Outcome

An objective measure of treatment outcome is essential, both in clinical and research settings. Outcome is a continual process and includes not only an assessment of seizure control, but also consideration of side effects and quality of life. A number of barriers to effective evaluation may be present. Information will, by necessity, be largely inferred from patients with limited communication skills and may be subject to "diagnostic overshadowing." A multidisciplinary approach will be required in most cases to obtain high-quality data, as many patients will have multiple caregivers in a variety of settings, all requiring guidance to produce accurate recordings. Espie and colleagues[16] described a three-tiered approach to the assessment of epilepsy treatment in persons with ID. The first involves the use of measures defining the individual; this may include etiology and seizure syndrome as well as use of assessment tools such as the Aberrant Behavior Checklist[17] and Adaptive Behavior Scale[18] in the evaluation of variables such as behavior and baseline functional ability. Measures that are sensitive to change are required to estimate response to treatment. Documentation of seizure description and frequency in the form of a diary is a well-recognized clinical tool. The Liverpool Seizure Severity Scale has been adapted for use in the intellectually disabled. Again, scales such as the Aberrant Behavior Checklist may be helpful in quantifying behavioral change; for an overall impression of general well-being the Epilepsy and Learning Disability Quality of Life Scale[19] may be beneficial. Finally, Espie advocates consideration of the effect of the patient's epilepsy upon their caregivers. A variety of scales, such as the Caregiver Strain Index, Hospital Anxiety and Depression Scale, or Beck Depression Inventory,[20]may be employed. They range from general quality of life measures to the more disorder-specific. The Glasgow Epilepsy Outcome Scale[21] has the obvious advantages of its specific design for the population concerned but also includes different scales for use by family and caregivers, thus recognizing that perceptions may differ. The scale comprises four subsections: concerns regarding seizures, treatment, caring, and social impact. Alternatively, a qualitative interview with caregivers or family can potentially add a different dimension to the assessment of outcome and may highlight factors left unexplored by quantitative analysis.

Conclusion

Antiepileptic medication is the mainstay of treatment for individuals with ID who have epilepsy. Appropriate skilled application should lead to reducing the inequality in health experienced by this population. Professionals in a position of treating this population should recognize and acquire the appropriate knowledge and competencies necessary to deliver such skilled use of treatments.

References

1. Baxter HA. (1999) Falls and fractures in a population with learning disability. 10th International Roundtable in Aging and Intellectual Disabilities. Geneva, Switzerland.
2. Morgan G, Scheepers M, Kerr M. (2001) Mortality in patients with intellectual disability and epilepsy. Curr Opin Psychiatr 14: 471–475.

3. Chadwick D, Reynolds EH. (1985) When do epileptic patients need treatment? Starting and stopping medication. Br Med J 290: 1885–1888.
4. Berg AT, Shinnar S. (1991) The risk of seizure recurrence following a first unprovoked seizure—a quantitative review. Neurology 41: 965–972.
5. Kwan P, Brodie MJ. (2001) The effectiveness of first antiepileptic drug. Epilepsia 42: 1255–1260.
6. Biraben A, Allain H, Scarabin JM, et al. et al. (2000) Exacerbations of juvenile myoclonic epilepsy with lamotrigine. Neurology 55: 1758.
7. Deckers CLP. (2002) The place of polytherapy in the early treatment of epilepsy. CNS Drugs 16: 155–163.
8. MRC Antiepileptic Drug Withdrawal Group. (1991) Randomised study of antiepileptic drug withdrawal in patients in remission. Lancet 337: 1175–1180.
9. Motte J, Trevathen E, Barrera MN, et al. et al. (1997) Lamotrigine for generalised seizures associated with the Lennox-Gastaut syndrome. N Engl J Med 337: 1807–1812.
10. Sachdeo R, Kugler S, Wenger E, et al. et al. (1996) Topiramate in Lennox-Gastaut syndrome. Epilepsia 37: 118.
11. Kerr M, Baker G, Brodie MD. (2005) A randomised double-blind, placebo controlled trial of topiramate in adults with epilepsy and intellectual disability: Impact on seizures, severity and quality of life. Epilepsy Behav 7: 472–480.
12. Crawford P, Brown S, Kerr M. (2001) A randomised open-label study of gabapentin and lamotrigine in adults with learning disability and resistant epilepsy. Seizure. 10:107–115.
13. Kelly K, Stephen LJ, Brodie MJ. (2004) Levetiracetam for people with mental retardation and refractory epilepsy. Epilepsy Behav 5: 878–883.
14. Collacott RA, Dignon A, Hauk A, et al. (1989) Clinical and therapeutic monitoring of epilepsy in a mental handicap unit. Br J Psychiatr 155: 522–525.
15. Alvarez N. (1989) Discontinuation of antiepileptic medications in patients with developmental disability and a diagnosis of epilepsy. Am J Ment Retard 93: 593–599.
16. Espie CA, KerrM, Paul A, et al. (1997) Learning disability and epilepsy, 2: A review of available outcome measures and position statement on development priorities. Seizure 6: 337–350.
17. Aman M, Singh N. (1983) Pharmacological intervention. In: Matson J, Mullick, J (eds.). Handbook of mental retardation. Pergamon, New York: 317–337.
18. Nihira K, Leyland H, Lambert N. (1993) Adaptive Behaviour Scales. American Association on Mental Retardation. Austin, Texas:
19. Jacoby A, Baker GA, Steen N, et al. (1996) The clinical course of epilepsy and its psychosocial correlates; findings from a UK community study. Epilepsia 37: 148–161.
20. Beck AT, SteerRA. (1997) The Beck Depression Inventory: Manual. The Psychological Corporation. San Antonio, Texas:
21. Espie CA, Watkins J, Duncan R, et al. (2001) Development and validation of the Glasgow Epilepsy Outcome Scale (GEOS); a new instrument for measuring concerns about epilepsy in people with mental retardation. Epilepsia 42: 1043–1051.

Chapter 8
Vagus Nerve Stimulation Therapy: An Intellectual Disabilities Perspective

V. P. Prasher, E. Furlong, and L. Weerasena

Introduction

Numerous studies have now been published confirming the high prevalence of epilepsy in people with intellectual disabilities (ID).[1-3] McDermott and colleagues[3] compared the rates of epilepsy between ID and non-ID groups living in the community. The non-LD group had an epilepsy prevalence rate of 1%. The prevalence of epilepsy within the LD group was 13% for cerebral palsy, 13.6% for Down syndrome (DS), 25.4% for autism, 25.5% for mental retardation, and 40% for adults with both cerebral palsy and ID. Further, the researchers found that during the decades of adulthood, the prevalence of epilepsy declined for those with cerebral palsy and ID. The prevalence of epilepsy increased with advancing years for adults with DS and autism. For each decade, the prevalence of epilepsy was higher in the ID group compared to the non-ID group.

A significant proportion of persons with ID will have intractable epilepsy. Antiepileptic drugs (AEDs) remain the principal form of management for intractable epilepsy with up to 40% of individuals on polytherapy.[4-5] However, poor seizure control may still be evident, leading to the consideration of alternative treatments. The principal alternative form of treatment is psychosurgery, but this is not readily accessible to persons with ID. Vagus nerve stimulation (VNS) therapy has the potential to be the main practical and efficacious treatment alternative to AEDs for individuals with ID who suffer from intractable epilepsy. To date there is very limited information specifically focused on the role of VNS Therapy to treat epilepsy in the ID population. This review chapter examines the role of VNS Therapy in persons with ID.

Background

In 1985 Dr. Jacob Zabara proposed that electrical stimulation of the vagus nerve had potential benefits in seizure prevention.[6] This hypothesis was based on observations from animal studies investigating the effects of VNS on electroencephalogram

V.P. Prasher, M.P. Kerr (eds.) *Epilepsy and Intellectual Disabilities*,
DOI: 10.1007/978-1-84800-259-3_8, © Springer Science+Business Media, LLC 2008

(EEG) recordings. Vagus nerve stimulation was found to induce EEG synchronization, EEG desynchronization, and REM and slow wave sleep in animals, depending on the different stimulus parameters.[7-8] As epileptic seizures are characterized by paroxysmal, abnormal synchronicity of the EEG, it was postulated that VNS could prevent seizure activity by desynchronizing the electrical activity of the brain.[6] Subsequently, animal experiments confirmed the anticonvulsant efficacy of VNS[9,10] and led to the development of an implantable VNS device by Cyberonics, Inc. (Houston, TX) for use in the treatment of patients with pharmacoresistant epilepsy.

The first actual vagus nerve stimulator was implanted in a patient with epilepsy in 1988.[11] Following open and randomized controlled trials (see Binnie[12] for review) VNS Therapy was approved in Europe in 1994 and in United States in1997 for use as an adjunctive therapy in reducing the frequency of seizures in patients whose epileptic disorder is dominated by partial seizures (with or without secondary generalization) or generalized seizures which are refractory to antiepileptic medications.

Vagus nerve stimulation therapy has dramatically changed the management of refractory epilepsy. It is now the most widely used nonpharmacological treatment and has been reported to be beneficial in reducing seizures, preventing seizures soon after VNS Therapy has been initiated; in reducing long-term seizure frequency, and improving quality of life. To date, over 20,000 patients have now had VNS implants for refractory seizures.

The VNS Therapy System™

The main component of the VNS Therapy System™ consists of a titanium-encased pulse generator (Figure 8.1) that delivers mild automatic intermittent electrical stimuli to the cervical portion of the left vagus nerve via a bipolar lead (the left vagus nerve has less cardiac regulation and therefore is used rather than the right vagus nerve). The pulse generator contains a battery and programmable computer chips. The stimulus is transmitted via the vagus nerve to the brain. The appropriate settings for the stimulation are determined by a telemetric wand (Figure 8.1), which is held over the pulse generator and controlled by computer software. Patients and/or caregivers can control the degree of stimulation (and side effects) by a hand-held magnet (Figure 8.1).

There have been improvements in VNS design and in the duration battery life of the pulse generator since the first commercially available model. The current device, model 102 (6.9 mm, weight 25g), is less bulky than the original NCP 100 model, resulting in a better cosmetic result following implantation and longer battery life. Depending on stimulus parameters and use, the pulse generator can now run for 6 to 11 years. However, once the battery is depleted, the entire pulse generator must be removed and replaced. The implantation procedure takes approximately one hour and is usually carried out under general anesthesia so as to limit the risk

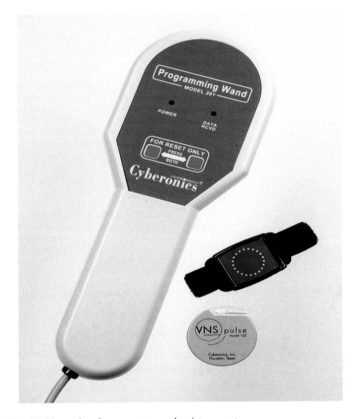

Fig. 8.1 Hand-held wand, pulse generator, and wrist magnet

of intraoperative seizures, which could result in damage to the vagus nerve or surrounding structures. Occasionally implants are inserted in awake patients using local anesthesia.

The surgical procedure requires a transverse incision on the left side of the neck, followed by careful dissection to expose the carotid sheath. The vagus nerve lies within the sheath between the carotid artery and the internal jugular vein. A subcutaneous pocket for the pulse generator is created over the fascia of the pectoral muscle via an incision in the left anterior axillary fold (approximately 8cm below the left clavicle). A tunneling tool is used to create a subcutaneous tract connecting the two incision sites. The bipolar lead is then introduced along the tunnel toward the vagus nerve. The lead makes contact with the nerve via terminal helical electrodes that are gentle wrapped around the vagus nerve and anchored in place. The other end of the lead is connected to the pulse generator and the system and lead are tested. The pulse generator is then placed in the subcutaneous pocket and the two sites are closed (see Figure 8.2).

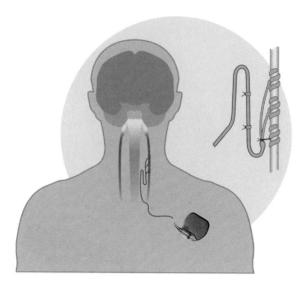

Fig. 8.2 Insertion of VNS. Electrodes wrapped around left vagus nerve. Electrical impulses sent up nerve to brain

The device can be activated immediately after implantation, but this may be delayed for two weeks. This delay allows time for postoperative recovery and any postoperative pain to diminish before adding the potential discomfort of VNS Therapy. The generator is then programmed to deliver intermittent stimulation at parameters selected from software installed on a laptop or palmtop computer. This information is transferred from computer to pulse generator via the programming telemetry wand placed over the chest wall. Programmable parameters include the output current, on-time (during which a train of stimulation is fired), off-time (during which no stimulation occurs), frequency and pulse width, magnet current output, magnet pulse width, and magnet activation time. The parameters can be adjusted over time according to individual response and tolerance. Additional stimulation can be initiated by placing a magnet over the generator for a few seconds. This can be carried out during an aura or seizure in an attempt to abort or shorten it or, postictally, to shorten the postictal period. The magnet can be used to deactivate the pulse generator. This may be necessary in the event that the patient is experiencing side effects of VNS Therapy or a malfunction is suspected.

Mechanism of Action

The exact mechanism of action of VNS Therapy in reducing seizure activity remains uncertain, although awareness of the anatomical and neurophysiological function of the left vagus nerve aids our understanding.[13,14] The left vagus nerve is the X cranial nerve and consists of approximately 80% afferent fibers and 20% efferent fibers.[15] The cell bodies of the efferent fibers are located in the nucleus ambiguus (NA) and the dorsal motor nucleus (DMN). Projections from the NA innervate striated muscles of the larynx, pharynx, and esophagus. Fibers from the DMN provide parasympathetic innervation to the heart, lungs, and gastrointestinal tract and influence heart rate, gastric secretions, and peristalsis. The afferent fibers transmit visceral sensory information to the central nervous system (CNS) from the heart, aorta, lungs, and gastrointestinal tract. They originate in the nodose ganglion and project primarily to the nucleus of the solitary tract (NTS) in the medulla oblongata. The NTS has direct and indirect connections to numerous areas of the brain, many of which are implicated in epileptogenesis.[16]. Through these pathways, stimulation of the vagus nerve may influence brain activity and therefore seizure discharge.

It remains unclear which of the many pathways are implicated in the therapeutic action of VNS Therapy. The locus coelreus (LC) and raphe nucleus (RN) both receive connections from the NTS and appear to be important in the anticonvulsant effect of VNS. Animal studies have demonstrated that bilateral lesions in these areas ameliorate the seizure-suppressing effects of VNS Therapy.[17] This suggests that noradrenaline and serotonin, neurotransmitters released by the LC and RN respectively, may mediate the anticonvulsant effect of VNS.[18]

Neurochemical studies investigating changes in cerebrospinal fluid (CSF) amino acid and neurotransmitter metabolites following VNS Therapy have shown increased concentrations in 5-hydroxyindoleatic acid and HMA, metabolites of serotonin and dopamine, respectively. Raised CSF GABA and glycine concentrations have also been demonstrated. It remains unclear if such changes play a role in the mechanism of action of VNS Therapy.[19,20]

Functional neuroimaging techniques have been used to observe the acute and chronic changes in cerebral blood flow (CBF) resulting from VNS Therapy. Changes in blood flow are thought to reflect alterations in synaptic activity. Such studies aid an understanding of the effects of VNS on brain activity levels and therefore may be important in developing an understanding of the mechanism of action of VNS Therapy. Studies of CBF in humans have produced conflicting results, although many demonstrate changes in the thalamus.[21,22]

Studies observing the effect of VNS on human EEG have produced inconsistent results. Some studies have confirmed the EEG benefits of VNS seen in animal studies in humans, where interictal epileptiform discharges were reduced, synchronization occurred, and a decrease in spike and wave activity was seen.[23,24] Others have failed to demonstrate VNS-induced suppression of interictal epileptic activity.[20,25]

Clinical Efficacy of VNS Therapy

A consensus of publishedstudies based on a mixed sample of individuals with and without ID has demonstrated the benefits of VNS Therapy.[13,16,26] Initially pilot studies showed the short-term benefit of VNS Therapy in refractory epilepsy.[11,23,27,28]

Uthman and colleagues[28] reported findings from two single-blind studies (designated EO1 and EO2) that treated 14 patients (no information given about IQ status). The mean reduction in seizure frequency after 14 to 35 months was 46.6%. Five (35.7%) individuals had a reduction of at least 50% seizure frequency. Vonck and colleagues[26] prospectively assessed 131 patients treated with VNS Therapy. The mean age of the patients was 32 years, and the mean duration of refractory epilepsy was 22 years. The mean reduction in monthly seizure frequency was 55%. Seven percent were free of seizures, 50% had a seizure frequency reduction of more than 50%, and 21% were nonresponders.

A number of randomized controlled studies have been reported,[29–31] confirming the findings from the earlier studies, which were more susceptible to investigator bias. The Vagus Nerve Stimulation Study Group[29] performed a multicenter RCT in 114 patients randomized to receive 14 weeks of high-level or low-level stimulation using a blinded parallel study design. No information was given regarding ID status. Mean reduction in seizure frequency was seen in both groups (24.5% for "high" group and 6.1% for "low" group. Thirty-one percent of the "high" group had a reduction of 50% or more seizure frequency.

The long-term benefits of VNS Therapy have been reported.[32–35] Morris and colleagues[33] evaluated the results of long-term open-label treatment of 440 patients with refractory epilepsy with VNS Therapy from five clinical trials. No information was given regarding ID status. A 50% seizure reduction occurred in 36.8% of patients at one year, in 43.2% at two years, and 42.7% at three years. Alexopoulos and colleagues[35] reviewed VNS data for 46 patients. The median age at implantation was 12.1 (range 2.3–17.9) years and the median duration of epilepsy 8.0 (1.9–16.9) years. Seizure frequency reduction in the range of 60% was observed at one, two, and three years post VNS. Overall long-term studies suggest that the efficacy of VNS Therapy is maintained over time.

Children

Although no RCT has investigated VNS Therapy exclusively in children, a number of studies do support the use of VNS Therapy for refractory seizures in children.[36–41] Parker and colleagues,[36] in a review of 15 children (majority with ID) implanted for at least one year, found four had a >50% reduction and two had a >50% increase in seizure frequency. Helmers and colleagues,[42] in a six-center retrospective study, reviewed data from 125 patients initially seen (39% with ID). The average seizure frequency was reduced by 36.1% at three months and 44.7% at six months. Rychlicki and colleagues[41] investigated the clinical efficacy, safety, and neuropsychological effects of VNS in 34 children (mean age 11.5 years) with drug-resistant epilepsy. Mean follow-up was 30.8 months. Mean reduction in total seizures was 39% at 3 months, 38% at 6 months, 49% at 12 months, 61% at 24 months and 71% at 36 months. Significantly better results were obtained in partial epilepsy, with and without drop attacks, than in Lennox-Gastaut syndrome – three patients being seizure-free. No operative morbidity was reported. Side effects were minor and transient – the most common were voice alteration and coughing during stimulation.

Although further controlled studies are necessary, available information would suggest that in children with ID and with intractable epilepsy, VNS Therapy is safe and effective.

Intellectual Disability Population

Few studies investigating the effects of VNS in persons with ID only have been reported (Table 8.1). Often patients with ID have been part of the overall study sample (above studies). Andriola and Vitale[46] undertook a retrospective review of 21 mild-severe ID patients who had VNS Therapy (age range 3–56 years). Sixty-eight percent had a greater than 50% reduction in seizure frequency at six months. There were no major adverse events. Further information is needed regarding the role of VNS Therapy to treat epilepsy in adults with ID.

VNS in Specific Learning-Disabled Persons

Landau-Kleffner Syndrome and Autism

Landau-Kleffner syndrome (LKS) is a rare childhood neurological disorder charac-terized by gradual or sudden loss of ability to comprehend or express spoken lan-guage. Children develop LKS between three and nine years of age, and approximately 80% of these children experience seizures. Park[48] analyzed retro-spective data from the VNS Therapy patient outcome registry (Cyberonics, Inc; Houston, TX, USA). Six patients (mean age at implantation 10.3 ± 4.2 years) with LKS were identified. Among the LKS patients, three patients at six months experi-enced at least a 50% reduction in seizure frequency as compared with baseline. Physicians reported quality-of-life improvements in all areas assessed for at least three of the six children. Further studies are necessary to demonstrate the potential benefits of VNS Therapy on seizures and language.

Autism

Autism is a pervasive developmental disorder characterized by abnormalities in communication, social interaction, and by restricted repetitive activities. This con-dition was first described by Kanner,[49] who named it infantile autism. About 25%

Table 8.1 Studies of VNS Therapy in study group including persons with intellectual disabilities.

Study	No. of patients	Severity of ID	Age range	Gender (M/F)	Findings
Majoie et al. [93]	16	Moderate or mild mental handicap	7–18 years	13/3	50% reduction in seizure frequency in 25% of patients
					Mean reduction in seizure frequency per patient of 26.9% Better outcome with higher mental age
Aldenkamp et al. [44]	16	Mental age given	6–19 years	13/3	Average reduction in seizure frequency of 26.9% after 6 months. Improvement in mental age, independent behavior and mood for some children.
Nagarajam et al. [45]	16	9 severe, 4 moderate, 3 mild	3–17 years	9/7	50% reduction in seizure frequency in 62.5% of patients. 90% reduction in seizure frequency in 25% of patients
Parker et al. [36]	15	Most with ID	5–16 years	—	50% reduction in seizure frequency in 27% of patients but 50% increase in 14%
Andriola and Vitale [46]	20	3 mild and 17 moderate or severe	3–56 years	17/3	68% of patients had 50% or more reduction in seizures after 6 months
Hornig et al. [47]	19	15 had ID	4–19 years	12/7	50% reduction in seizure frequency in 53% of patients
					90% reduction in seizure frequency in 32% of patients

of autistic children normally develop seizures about the time of adolescence. Park,[48] in his report of analysis of retrospective data from the VNS Therapy patient outcome registry (Cyberonics, Inc; Houston, TX, USA) for 59 persons with autism, found that 58% of the patients with autism (mean age of implantation12.4 ± 7.7 years) experienced at least a 50% reduction in seizure frequency at 12 months. Improvements in all areas of quality of life (QoL) monitored were reported for most patients, particularly for alertness (76% at 12 months). The physicians reported more than half of the patients to be better in the areas of achievement (53%), mood (61%), postictal period (58%), and seizure clustering (53%). Interestingly, the authors noticed that the improvements in QoL were independent from the effect of VNS therapy on seizures. A limitation to these QoL analyses is that they were retrospectively made and no validated QoL scale was used. Research studies are ongoing to determine the role of VNS Therapy in autism.

Lennox-Gastaut Syndrome

Lennox-Gastaut syndrome and infantile spasms are rare childhood epilepsy syndromes characterized by intractable epilepsy. Up to 50% of children with infantile spasm develop LGS. Infantile spasms are often referred to as West's syndrome, which consists of a triad of signs and symptoms such as spasms (seizure type), hypsarrhythmias (the classic EEG), and mental retardation. Variations of this syndrome are not uncommon.William Lennox first described the clinical features of an "epileptic encephalopathy" with multiple seizure types and ID. Later on Lennox and Davies redescribed a symptomatic triad of:

1. Slow spike and wave on EEG
2. Mental deficiency
3. Three seizure types which are now referred to as atypical absence attacks

In 1966 Gastaut expanded and verified the original observations by Lennox and Gastaut. The following are current criteria for the syndrome:

1. Multiple seizures including absence seizures and catatonic seizures
2. EEG with slow spike and wave (C 2.5 Hz) and bursts of fast rhythms
3. Static encephalopathy and learning disability

About 5% of childhood epilepsy can be categorized as LGS. Up to 10% of children with LGS die within the first 11 years of their life.

A number of studies have investigated VNS Therapy in persons with LGS — usually as part of a larger cohort of ID persons.[41,47,50,51] The short-term benefits of VNS Therapy to persons with LGS remain controversial. Hornig and colleagues[47] found 90% reduction in seizures for five of six children, whereas Rychlicki and colleagues[41] found children with LGS did less well than those with partial epilepsy. Hosain and colleagues[52] studied 13 patients with LGS. The median age of the patients was 13 years, and a median of 6 AEDs (range, 4 to 12) were used prior to VNS Therapy implantation. At six months of follow-up, 3 of 13 patients had a greater than 90% reduction in number of seizures, 2 had a greater than 75% seizure reduction, and 1 had a greater than 50% seizure reduction. In total, 6 of the 13 patients (46%) were responders to VNS Therapy. Of the remaining 7 patients, 6 had at least 25% seizure reduction and only one had no improvement in number of seizures.

In 2001, Aldenkamp and colleagues[44] reported the long-term effects of VNS on children with LGS. They reported a modest effect on seizure frequency (20.6% at 24/12) but only minor changes in behavioral outcomes such as independency, behavioral problems, and moods. However, none of these changes were statistically significant, and the degree of ID was a negative prognostic factor for VNS treatment. Ben-Menachem and colleagues[53] assessed the long-term efficacy of VNS Therapy in 64 refractory epilepsy patients. Among those, 8 patients were diagnosed with LGS. Five of these LGS patients had undergone previous callosotomy. Five-eighths (62.5%) of the LGS patients treated with VNS Therapy were responders in all seizure types. The seizures that best responded to the treatment were the generalized tonic-clonic seizures and absences. For 2 of the 5 responders, the atonic seizures also decreased significantly.

Most of the studies in patients with LGS are conducted in a restricted number of patients. These studies are reporting seizure reductions in patients with LGS, and these range from 27% to 58% at 6 months postimplantation or longer. The patients' characteristics, the duration of the follow-up and the parameters settings might be elements explaining differences in the figures. Further research investigating VNS Therapy in a large sample of LGS patients only is still required.

Ring Chromosome 20 Syndrome

Ring chromosome 20 is a rare disorder characterized by ring-shaped chromosome 20, learning disabilities, seizures that are generally resistant to AED, behavioral problems, and dysmorphic features. Ring 20 (r[20]) syndrome was first described by Atkins and colleagues,[54] and more than 30 cases have been reported so far. The majority of cases describe severe intractable seizures, but some very rare cases are reported without seizures, probably due to phenotype variation. Ring chromosomes are caused by fusion of two arms of a chromosome. The formation of the ring chromosome is associated with deletions of the telomeric regions. A deletion of the short arm in chromosome 20 does not cause epilepsy, but the terminal deletion of the long arm in the 20q13 region results in epilepsy. Two other epileptic syndromes are also associated with a gene located in this region, namely autosomal dominant nocturnal frontal lobe epilepsy or benign neonatal convulsions. The severity of the syndromes is associated with the size of the deletion.

Chawla and colleagues[55] described success with VNS Therapy for intractable seizures associated with ring 20 chromosome syndrome in a girl of six years of age. She tried unsuccessfully with variations of AED and a ketogenic diet. This patient remained seizure free at nine months of follow up and became more social and achieved new developmental milestones. However, Alpman and colleagues[56] did not have similar success with their reported patient with ring 20 chromosome disorder, who was severely affected with epilepsy that did not respond to AEDs. He was implanted with a VNS Therapy system at the age of 11 years. In the first six months his seizure frequency decreased by approximately 50%, but six months later the tonic seizures during sleep and secondary generalized seizures continued one to three times per day despite the elevation of the output and magnet currents to 2.5 and 3mV. A corpus callosotomy was therefore performed at the age of 13 years. Unfortunately the patient remained uncontrolled and his behavioral problems became even more prominent.

A recent case was reported by Parr and colleagues[57] in a patient aged nine years old. This patient began to experienced seizures at five years of age. The seizures were taking various forms: upward deviation of the eyes, associated with episodes of confusion lasting up to one hour; arrest of activity with upward deviation of the eyes; eyelid flickering; and loss of posture, followed by postictal sleep. The patient had been treated with several antiepileptic medications, including sodium valproate, lamotrigine, clobazam, prednisolone, and leviteracetam. In addition, while on clobazam, rapid regression of skills occurred, resulting in complete loss of language and ambulation. At the age of eight, the patient was implanted with a VNS Therapy system. Initially, the patient responded well to the therapy with a reduction in the number of seizures and reacquisition of some previously lost skills, including ambulation. Improvements were also reported in eye contact and social smiling. Those improvements were noticed despite a continuation of the generalized tonic-clonic seizures (GTCS) and absence seizures. To improve the seizure control, the output current was increased to 2.5mA, which led to a worsening of the seizures. The reduction of the current to 2.25mA led to a gradual improvement with a return to the previous improved state. At the time of publication, the patient was on a combination of leviteracetam monotherapy and VNS Therapy. He remained ambulant, and seizures were confined to occasional nocturnal episodes.

Tuberous Sclerosis

Tuberous sclerosis (TSC) is a rare genetic disease that causes benign tumors to grow in the brain and on other vital organs such as the kidneys and heart. It commonly affects the central nervous system. In addition to the benign tumors that frequently occur in TSC, other common symptoms include seizures, mental retardation, behavior problems, and skin abnormalities. Tuberous sclerosis may be present at birth, but full symptoms may take some time to develop. The disorder is due to a mutation in the TSC1 or the TSC2 gene. Epilepsy is the most common presenting symptom in TSC as 80–90% of the patients with TSC will develop epilepsy.[58]

Parain and colleagues[59] studied the outcome of VNS Therapy in children with tuberous sclerosis complex who had medically refractory epilepsy. It was an open label retrospective, multicenter study looking at records of all children treated with VNS in five pediatric epilepsy centers. All patients were studied at least for six months. Ten patients were identified. The researchers found that nine children had at least 50% reduction in seizure frequency and over half had a 90% or greater reduction in seizure frequency. Increased alertness was also reported. Further studies are necessary to confirm that VNS Therapy is effective and well tolerated in patients with tuberous sclerosis complex.

Rett Syndrome

Rett syndrome is often a sporadic disorder occurring in 1 in 10,000 to 23,000 girls worldwide. Rett syndrome is associated with profound mental and motor disability, and in 90% of the cases it is associated with a mutation in the methyl-c9G binding protein 2 gene (MECP2).

Wilfong and colleagues[60] reported a case series of seven females with Rett syndrome who were implanted with a VNS Therapy system. The follow-up was minimum 12 months after implantation. The median age was nine years, and they had experienced seizures for a median time of six years. The patients had tried and failed two treatments with antiepileptic drugs (range, 2 to 8) before undergoing VNS Therapy implantation.

After 12 months of therapy, six of the seven patients had experienced at least 50% seizure reduction. Four of these seven responders even recorded seizure reductions greater than 90%. No difference was seen in MECP2-positive or -negative patients.

Adverse Effects and Safety

The adverse effects of VNS Therapy can be considered in the following categories: those related to surgical implantation of the device, stimulation-related, and serious adverse events (Table 8.2).

Surgically Related

Postoperative infections occur in approximately 3–6% of patients. Such infections usually respond to oral antibiotics and rarely require removal of the device or leads.[31,34] Pain is common in the postoperative period but diminishes with time as the implant wound heals.[61] Left cord paralysis and lower facial weakness have been

Table 8.2 Significant Adverse Effects of VNS Therapy

Perioperative	Stimulation-Related	Serious
Infection	Voice alteration (hoarseness)	Bradycardia
Postoperative pain	Cough	Asystole
Fluid accumulation around site	Dyspnea	Aspiration
	Muscle pain	Damage to carotid artery
Vocal cord weakness	Paresthesias	Vagus nerve paralysis
	Headache	
	Hypersalivation	
	Aspiration	
	Ataxia	
	Dyspepsia	
	Insomnia	
	Nausea	
	Vomiting	
	Somnolence	

reported following surgery.[31,62,63] Such adverse events are rare and have declined as experience with the surgical technique increases. Bradycardia and asystole have been reported as rare events during intraoperative testing of the system,[64,65] but no deaths have resulted. Asystole has not been recorded outside the operating theater.[64]

Side Effects

The most common side effects result from intermittent stimulation of the vagal innervation of the larynx. Such adverse events occur during trains of stimulation and include voice alteration (30–64%), cough (43–45%), throat discomfort (25–35%), throat paresthesia (18–25%), and dyspnea (11–25%). Other less common side effects have been reported, such as muscle pain, chest pain, headache, chronic diarrhea, Horner syndrome, psychotic episodes, nausea and vomiting.[66–68]

Swallowing difficulties and aspiration have been noted in children undergoing VNS, but conflicting reports have been published. Results from one study found that a sample of children with severe motor and mental impairment were at increased risk from aspiration while being fed during stimulation.[69] Sudden unexplained death in epilepsy (SUDEP) has been reported in persons receiving VNS Therapy[70]; however, the incidence is comparable to that in persons with intractable epilepsy but not receiving VNS.

Few patients discontinue treatment as a result of adverse events. Most of the stimulation-related side effects diminish with time or alteration of stimulation parameters. Further, the revision or removal of the stimulating electrodes following long-term therapy does not lead to any adverse events intraoperatively or postoperatively.[71]

Vagus nerve stimulation therapy lacks side effects such as sedation, psychomotor slowing, and weight gain that are experienced with some AEDs. It does not alter blood biochemistry, cardiac and pulmonary function tests, or AED serum concentrations, so it can be used safely in combination with pharmacological treatments.[34]

Serious Adverse Events

In the preapproval E-03 study, the safety of VNS Therapy was analyzed by Ramsay and colleagues.[72] No serious adverse events were reported in association with normal VNS Therapy. One patient's experienced extreme pain, hoarseness, and left vocal cord paralysis due to a short circuit in the generator. Some symptoms persisted up to one year after the incident.

The mortality rates of persons undergoing VNS Therapy have been reported to be comparable to those of similar groups of individuals who have intractable epilepsy but have been treated with standard AEDs.[70] The incidence of SUDEP was not significantly increased with VNS Therapy. During implantation, transient asystole has been reported in several patients but with no serious or permanent sequelae.

VNS Therapy and Neurological Investigations

Electroencephalogram Changes and VNS

A number of studies observing electroencephalogram (EEG) recordings in both humans and animals undergoing VNS have been reported.[50,73,74] Most animal studies have demonstrated the suppression of both ictal and interictal eplieptiform EEG findings during stimulation. Kuba and colleagues[73] studied 15 patients, all treated with VNS Therapy for at least six months. For each individual the interictal epileptiform discharges (IED) were counted at the baseline period (BP), the stimulation period (SP), six interstimulation periods (IP), and the prestimulation period (PP). The number of IEDs at BP and PP were compared with the number of IED at SP and IP. This study was carried out by the Bruno Epilepsy Centre in the Czech Republic. Of the 15 patients 4 were women and 11 were men. They had had epilepsy for an average of 24.2 ± 9.5 years and were aged 36.0 ± 7.1 years.

After implantation, parameters of chronic VNS Therapy were applied. There were eight patients with temporal lobe epilepsy and seven patients with extratemporal epilepsy. Previous surgery for epilepsy had been performed in seven patients. Interestingly, in this study, the highest reduction of IED occurred during the SP as compared with the BP in 14/15 patients (93%) and in 12/15 (80%) patients as compared with the PP. From this point of view their study contrasts other data from similar human studies.

The reduction in the number of IED during SP was significantly higher in patients who had experienced positive clinical results with VNS Therapy. In interpreting the results the authors added that the positive effects of acute stimulation in suppressing the interictal graphoelements probably predict candidates who will show superior efficacy if VNS stimulation is prescribed. They also postulate that the mechanism of desynchronization of epileptiform activity by VNS Therapy is the probable mechanism of action.

Functional Magnetic Resonance Imaging (fMRI) and VNS

Few studies have investigated functional brain changes in persons undergoing VNS Therapy.[75–77] Narayanan and colleagues[75] studied the short-term effects of VNS Therapy on brain activation and cerebral blood flow by using functional magnetic resonance imaging (fMRI).They studied five patients with a mean age of 35.4 years — three women and two men. All five patients tolerated fMRI successfully.

Blood flow increases were seen in the dorsocentral medulla, right post central gryus, right thalamus, bilateral insular cortices, hypothalami, and bilateral inferior cerebellar regions. Significant decreases in blood flow were observed in the amygdala, hippocampi, and posterior cingulated gyri. The researchers proposed that thalamic and insular cortical areas of the brain could play a role in modulating cerebral activity during seizure activity.

In contrast, in a further study, also of a limited number of participants (N = 4), Sucholeiki and colleagues[76] found that fMRI activation was seen in the left superior temporal gyrus, inferior frontal gyrus, medial portions of the superior frontal gryus, in the region of the supplementary motor cortex, and the posterior aspect of the middle frontal gyrus. Little activation was seen in the brainstem, thalamus, or basal ganglia. Liu and colleagues[77] found brain activation in the frontal and occipital lobes. Further research involving a larger number of subjects is required.

SPECT Brain Images and VNS Therapy Stimulation

Positron emission computerized tomography and single positron emission computerized tomography (SPECT) remain tools of further investigation of VNS Therapy. Reduced perfusion during stimulation in the ipsilateral brainstem, cingulate, amygdala, and hippocampus and contralateral thalamus has been reported.[78] Ring and colleagues[79] had earlier reported, in a study of seven subjects, relatively decreased activity in left and right medial thalamic regions. Such reports suggest that VNS may act either by modulating activity in the limbic and subcortical areas, which act as relay stations for seizure discharges.

Other Benefits of VNS Therapy

Two of the most significant secondary benefits of VNS Therapy are the reduction in drug and dosage of AEDs without loss of seizure control[80] and the cost benefits of VNS Therapy.[81–83] Boon and colleagues[82] reported a mean drop in hospital admission days (from 16 to 4 days/year) and a reduction in direct medical costs per patient.

Beneficial clinical effects beyond changes in seizure frequency have been observed. Malow and colleagues[84] found that in 16 patients treatment with low stimulus intensities improved daytime sleepiness and promoted alertness. The use of VNS Therapy to reduce morbid obesity,[85,86] improve memory,[87] improve treatment-resistant depression,[88] and to elevate mood[89–91] have been reported. Pilot studies investigating the role of VNS Therapy for Alzheimer's disease, obsessive-compulsive disorder, migraine headaches, and anxiety disorders are underway.

Conclusion

This chapter has reviewed the impact of VNS Therapy to treat partial-onset retractable epilepsy in individuals with ID. The ID population is arguably the largest population where VNS Therapy could have the most dramatic impact. Well over 20,000 patients have been implanted with the VNS Therapy system but limited clinical and research information is available exclusively relating to children and/or adults with ID. Many persons with ID have been part of limited research studies, but their findings have often not been reported separately. From available information, studies suggest that VNS Therapy has comparable efficacy to new antiepileptic drugs, is safe, well tolerated, and manageable. The long-term beneficial effects of VNS Therapy appear to be greater than standard anticonvulsant medication; clinical experience would suggest maximum benefit from VNS Therapy might not be apparent for at least one year.

Patients being put forward for VNS Therapy should be determined by their suitability for the procedure (type of seizure disorder, previous response to AEDs, health status, compliance with day-to-day use) and the likely benefits (e.g., quality of life, reduction in medication). Vagus nerve stimulation therapy should be recommended after the failure of three or four adequate trials of AEDs in persons with diagnosed partial or generalized epilepsy.

Many unanswered questions remain regarding the use of VNS Therapy in individuals with ID. These include (1) a need for randomized controlled clinical trials in persons with ID only, (2) further investigation of adverse effects in individuals with high comorbidity, (3) which factors determine a good response (e.g., severity of ID, etiology of ID, type of seizures), (4) impact on quality of life, and (5) the long-term effects.

Vagus nerve stimulation therapy has had a dramatic impact on the management of epilepsy generally. It has heralded a new era in the treatment of epilepsy and should also benefit individuals with ID.

References

1. Coulter DL. (1993) Epilepsy and mental retardation: An overview. Am J Ment Retard. 98: 1–11.
2. Bowley C, Kerr M. (2000) Epilepsy and intellectual disability. J Intellect Disabil Res 44: 529–543.
3. McDermott S, Moran R, Platt T, et al. (2005) Prevalence of epilepsy in adults with mental retardation and related disabilities in primary care. Am J Ment Retard 110: 48–56.
4. Espie CA, Gillies JB, Montgomery JM. (1990) Antiepileptic polypharmacy, psychosocial behaviour and locus of control orientation among mentally handicapped adults living in the community. J Ment Defic Res. 34: 351–360.
5. Singh BK, Towle PO. (1993) Antiepileptic drug status in adult outpatients with mental retardation. Am J Ment Retard 98: 41–46.
6. Zabara J. (1985) Peripheral control of hypersynchronous discharge in epilepsy. Electroencephal Clin Neurophysiol. 61: 162.
7. Zanchetti A, Wang SC, Moruzzi G. (1952) Effect of afferent vagal stimulation on the electroencephalogram of the cat in cerebral isolation. B Soc Ital Biol Sper. 28: 627–628.
8. Chase MH, Sterman MB, Clemente CD. (1966) Cortical and subcortical patterns of response to afferent vagal stimulation. Exper Neurol. 16: 36–49.
9. Woodbury DM, Woodbury JW. (1990) Effects of vagal stimulation on experimentally induced seizures in rats. Epilepsia 31: S7–s19.
10. Lockard JS, Congdon WC, DuCharme LL. (1990) Feasibility and safety of vagal stimulation in monkey model. Epilepsia 31: S20–s26.
11. Penry JK, Dean JC. (1990) Prevention of intractable partial seizures by intermittent vagal stimulation in humans: Preliminary results. Epilepsia 31: S40–s43.
12. Binnie CD. (2000) Vagus nerve stimulation for epilepsy: A review. Seizure 9: 161–169.
13. Vonck K, Laere K, Van Dedeurwaerdere ST, et al. et al. (2001) The mechanism of action of vagus nerve stimulation for refractory epilepsy. J Clin Neurophysiol 18: 394–401.
14. Henry TR. (2002) Therapeutic mechanisms of vagus nerve stimulation. Neurology. 59: S3–S14.
15. Rutecki P. (1990) Anatomical, physiological, and theoretical basis for the antiepileptic effect of vagus nerve stimulation. Epilepsia 31: S1–s6.
16. Boon P, Vonck K, Reuck J, et al. De et al. (2001) Vagus nerve stimulation for refactory epilepsy. Seizure 10: 448–455.
17. Krahl SE, Clark KB, Smith DC, et al. et al. (1998) Locus coeruleus lesions suppress the seizure-attenuating effects of vagus nerve stimulation. Epilepsia 39: 709–714.
18. Amar AP, Heck CN, DeGiorgio, CM, et al. et al. (1999). Experience with vagus nerve stimulation for intractable epilepsy: Some questions and answers. Neurol Med Chir (Tokyo) 39: 489–495.
19. Ben-Menachem E. (1996) Vagus nerve stimulation. Bailliere's Clin Neurol 5: 841–848.
20. Hammond EJ, Uthman BM, Reid SA, et al. et al. (1992) Electrophysiological studies of cervical vagus nerve stimulation in humans: I. EEG effects. Epilepsia 33: 1013–1020.
21. Henry TR. (1998) 10 most commonly asked questions about vagus nerve stimulation for epilepsy. Neurologist 39: 677–686.
22. Vonck K, Boon P, Laere K, et al. Van et al. (2000) Acute single photon emission computed tomographic study of vagus nerve stimulation in refractory epilepsy. Epilepsia 41: 601–609.
23. Olejnieczak PW, Fisch BJ, Carey M, et al. et al. (2001) The effect of vagus nerve stimulation on epileptiform activity recorded from hippocampal depth electrodes. Epilepsia 42: 423–429.

24. Koo B. (2001) EEG changes with vagus nerve stimulation. J Clin Neurophysiol 18: 434–441.
25. Salinsky MC, Burchiel KJ. (1993) Vagus nerve stimulation has no effect on awake EEG rhythms in humans. Epilepsia 34: 299–304.
26. Vonck K, Thadani V, Gilbert K, et al. (2004) Vagus nerve stimulation for refractory epilepsy: A transatlantic experience. J Clin Neurophysiol 21: 283–289.
27. Uthman BM., Wilder BJ, Hammond EJ, et al. (1990) Efficacy and safety of vagus nerve stimulation in patients with complex partial seizures. Epilepsia 31: S44–s50.
28. Uthman BM, Wilder BJ, Penry JK, et al. (1993) Treatment of epilepsy by stimulation of the vagus nerve. Neurology 43: 1338–1345.
29. The Vagus Nerve Stimulation Study Group. (1995) A randomized controlled trial of chronic vagus nerve stimulation for treatment of medically intractable seizures. Neurology 45: 224–230.
30. Amar AP, Heck CN, Levy ML, et al. (1998) An institutional experience with cervical vagus nerve trunk stimulation for medically refactory epilepsy: Rationale, technique, and outcome. Neurosurgery 43: 1265–1280.
31. Handforth A, DeGiorgio CM, Schachter, et al. (1998) Vagus nerve stimulation therapy for partial-onset seizures. Neurology 51: 48–55.
32. Salinsky MC, Uthman BM, Ristanovic RK, et al. (1996) The Vagus Nerve Stimulation Study Group. Vagus Nerve Stimulation for the Treatment of Medically Intractable Seizures. Arch Neurol 53: 1176–1180.
33. Morris GL, Mueller WM. The Vagus Nerve Stimulation Group E01–E05. (1999) Long-term treatment with vagus nerve stimulation in patients with refractory epilepsy. Neurology 53: 1731–1735.
34. DeGiorgio CM, Schachter SC, Handforth A, et al. (2000) Prospective long-term study of vagus nerve stimulation for the treatment of refactory seizures. Epilepsia. 41: 1195–1200.
35. Alexopoulos AV, Kotagal P, Loddenkemper T, et al. (2006) Long-term results with vagus nerve stimulation in children with pharmacoreresistant epilepsy. Seizure. 15: 491–503.
36. Parker APJ, Polkey CE, Binnie CD, et al. (1999) Vagal nerve stimulation in epileptic encephalopathies. Pediatrics 1003: 778–782.
37. Lundgren J, Amark P, Blennow G, et al. (1998) Vagus nerve stimulation in 16 children with refractory epilepsy. Epilepsia 39: 809–813.
38. Murphy JV, Pediatric VNS Study Group. (1999) Left vagal nerve stimulation in children with medically refractory epilepsy. J Pediatr 34: 563–566.
39. Frost M, Gates J, Helmers SL, et al. (2001) Vagus nerve stimulation in children with refactory seizures associated with Lennox-Gastaut syndrome. Epilepsia 42: 1148–1152.
40. Benifla M, Rutka JT, Logan W, et al. (2006). Vagal nerve stimulation for refractory epilepsy in children: Indications and experience at The Hospital for Sick Children. Child Nerv Syst 22: 1018–1026.
41. Rychlicki F, Zamponi N, Trignani R, et al. (2006) Vagus nerve stimulation: Clinical experience in drug-resistant pediatric epileptic patients. Seizure 15: 483–490.
42. Helmers SL, Wheless JW, Frost M, et al. (2001) J Child Neurol 16: 843–848.
43. Majoie HJM, Berfelo MW, Aldenkamp AP, et al. (2001) Vagus nerve stimulation in children with therapy-resistant epilepsy diagnosed as Lennox-Gastaut syndrome. J Clin Neurophysiol 18: 419–428.
44. Aldenkamp AP, Veerdonk SHA, Van de Majoie HJM, et al. et al. (2001) Effects of 6 months of treatment with vagus nerve stimulation on behavior in children with Lennox-Gastaut syndrome in an open clinical and nonrandomized study. Epilepsy Behav 2: 343–350.
45. Nagarajan L, Walsh NL, Gregory P, et al. (2002) VNS Therapy in clinical practice in children with refractory epilepsy. Acta Neurol Scand 105: 13–17.
46. Andriola MR, Vitale A. (2001) Vagus nerve stimulation in the developmentally disabled. Epilepsy Behav 2: 129–134.
47. Hornig GW, Murphy JV, Schallert G, et al. (1997) Left vagus nerve stimulation in children with refractory epilepsy: An update. South Med J 90: 484–488.

48. Park YD. (2003) The effects of vagus nerve stimulation therapy on patients with intractable seizures and either Landau-Kleffner syndrome or autism. Epilpesy Behav 4: 286–290.
49. Kanner L. (1943) Autistic disturbances of affective contact. Nervous Child 2: 217–250.
50. Casazza M, Avanzini G, Ferroli P, et al. (2006) Vagal nerve stimulation: Relationship between outcome and electroclinical seizure pattern. Seizure 15: 198–207.
51. Buoni S, Mariottini A, Pieri S, et al. (2004) Vagus nerve stimulation for drug-resistant epilepsy in children and young adults. Brain Dev 26: 158–163.
52. Hosain S, Nikalov B, Harden, C, et al. (2000). Vagus nerve stimulation treatment for Lennox-Gastaut syndrome. J Child Neurol 15: 509–512.
53. Ben-Menachem E, Hellstrom K, Waldton C. (1999) Evaluation of refractory epilepsy treated with vagus nerve stimulation for up to 5 years. Neurology 52: 1265–1267.
54. Atkins L, Miller, WL, Salam M. (1972) A ring-20 chromosome. J Med Genet 9: 377–380.
55. Chawla J, Sucholeiki R, Jones C, et al. (2002) Intractable epilepsy with ring chromosome 20 syndrome treated with vagal nerve stimulation: Case report and review of the literature. J Child Neurol 17: 778–780.
56. Alpman A, Serdaroglu G, Cogulu, O, et al. (2005) Ring chromosome 20 syndrome with intractable epilepsy. Dev Med Child Neurol 48: 80.
57. Parr JR, Pang K, Mollett A, et al. (2006) Epilepsy responds to vagus nerve stimulation in ring chromosome 20 syndrome. Dev Med Child Neurol 48: 80.
58. Thiele EA. (2004) Managing epilepsy in tuberous sclerosis complex. J Child Neurol 19: 680–686.
59. Parain D, Penniello MJ, Berquen, P. (2001) Vagal nerve stimulation in tuberous sclerosis complex patients. Pediatr Neurol 25: 213–216.
60. Wilfong AA, Schultz RJ. (2006) Vagus nerve stimulation for treatment of epilepsy in Rett syndrome. Dev Med Child Neurol 48: 683–686.
61. Matthews, K, Elijamel MS. (2003) Vagus nerve stimulation and refractory depression: Please can you switch me on doctor? Br J Psychiatr 183: 181–183.
62. Ben-Menachem E. (2001). Vagus nerve stimulation, side effects, and long term safety. (2001). J Clin Neurophysiol. 18: 415–418.
63. Lockard JS, Ojemann GA, Congdon WC, et al. (1979). Cerebellar stimulation in alumina-gel monkey model: inverse relationship between clinical seizures and EEG interictal bursts. Epilepsia 20: 223–234.
64. Tatum, WO, 4th, Moore DB, Stecker MM, et al. (1999) Ventricualr asystole during vagus nerve stimulation for epilepsy in humans. Neurology 52: 1267–1269.
65. Asconape JJ, Moore DD, Zipes DP, et al. (1999) Bradycardia and asystole with the use of vagus nerve stimulation for the treatment of epilepsy: A rare complication of intraoperative device testing. Epilepsia 40: 1452–1454.
66. Zalvan C, Sulica L, Wolf S, et al. (2003) Laryngopharyngeal dysfunction from the implant vagal nerve stimulator. Laryngoscope 113: 221–225.
67. Kersing W, Dejonckere PH, Aa, HE, et al. van deret al. (2002) Laryngeal and vocal changes during vagus nerve stimulation in epileptic patients. J Voice 16: 251–257.
68. Charous SJ, Kempster G, Manders, E, et al. (2001) The effect of vagal nerve stimulation on voice. Laryngoscope. 111: 2028–2031.
69. Lundgren J, Ekberg O, Olsson, R. (1998) Aspiration: A potential complication to vagus nerve stimulation. Epilepsia 39: 998–1000.
70. Annegers JF, Coan SP, Hauser WA, et al. (2000) Epilepsy, vagal nerve stimulation by the NCP system, all-cause mortality, and sudden, unexpected, unexplained death. Epilepsia 41: 549–553.
71. Espinosa J, Aiello MT, Naritoku DK. (1999) Revision and removal of stimulating electrodes following long-term therapy with the vagus nerve stimulator. Surg Neurol 51: 659–664.
72. Ramsay RE, Uthman BM, Augustinsson LE, et al. (1994). Vagus nerve stimulation for treatment of partial seizures: 2. Safety, side effects, and tolerability. First International Vagus Nerve Stimulation Study Group. Epilepsia 1994. 35: 627–636.

73. Kuba R, Guzaninova M, Brazdil M, et al. (2002) Effect of vagal nerve stimulation on interictal epileptiform discharges: A scalp EEG study. Epilepsia 43: 1181–1188.

74. Marrosu F, Santoni F, Puligheddu M, et al. (2005) Increase in 20–50 Hz (gamma frequencies) power spectrum and synchronization after chronic vagal nerve stimulation. Clin Neurophysiol 116: 2026–2036.

75. Narayanan JT, Watts R, Haddad N, et al. (2002) Cerebral activation during vagus nerve stimulation: A functional MR study. Epilepsia 43: 1509–1514.

76. Sucholeiki R, Alsaadi TM, Morris GL. (2002) fMRI in patients implanted with a vagal nerve stimulator. Seizure 11: 157–162.

77. Liu WC, Mosier K, Kalnin AJ, et al. (2003) BOLD f MRI activation induced by vagus nerve stimulation in seizure patients. J Neurol Neurosurg Psychiatr 74: 811–813.

78. Barnes A, Duncan R, Chisholm JA. (2003) Investigation into the mechanisms of vagus nerve stimulation for the treatment of intractable epilepsy, using 99mTc-HMPAO SPECT brain images. Eur J Nucl Med Mol Imaging 30: 301–305.

79. Ring HA, White S, Costa DC, et al. (2000) A SPECT study of the effect of vagal nerve stimulation on thalamic activity in patients with epilepsy. Seizure 9: 380–384.

80. Tatum WO, Johnson KD, Goff S, et al. (2001) Vagus nerve stimulation and drug reduction. Neurology 56: 561–563.

81. Jacoby A, Buck D, Baker G, et al. (1998) Uptake and costs of care for epilepsy: Findings from a U.K. regional study. Epilepsia 39: 776–786.

82. Boon P, Vonck K, D'Have M, et al. (1999) Cost-benefit of vagus nerve stimulation for refactory epilepsy. Acta Neurol Bel 99: 275–280.

83. Boon P, D'Have MD, Walleghem P, et al. Vanet al. (2002) Direct medical costs of refactory epilepsy incurred by three different treatment modalities: A prospective assessment. Epilepsia 43: 96–102.

84. Malow BA, Edwards J, Marzec M, et al. (2001) Vagus nerve stimulation reduces daytime sleepiness in epilepsy patients. Neurology 57: 879–884.

85. Roslin M, Kurian M. (2001) The use of electrical stimulation of the vagus nerve to treat morbid obesity. Epilepsy Behav. 2: S11–S16.

86. Sobocki J, Krolczyk G, Herman RM, et al. (2005) Influence of vagal nerve stimulation on food intake and body weight — results of experimental studies. J Physiol Pharmacol. 56: 27–33.

87. Clarke KB, Naritoku DK, Smith DC, et al. (1999). Enhanced recognition memory following vagus nerve stimulation in human subjects. Nature Neurosci 2: 94–98.

88. Sackeim HA, Keilp JG, Rush AJ, et al. (2001) The effects of vagus nerve stimulation on cognitive performance in patients with treatment-resistant depression. Neuropsy Neuropsy Be 14: 53–62.

89. Harden CL, Pulver MC, Ravdin LD, et al. (2000) A pilot study of mood in epilepsy patients treated with vagus nerve stimulation. Epilepsy Behav. 1: 93–99.

90. Hoppe C, Helmstaedter C, Scherrmann J, et al. (2001) Self-reported mood changes following 6 months of vagus nerve stimulation in epilepsy patients. Epilepsy Behav 2: 335–342.

91. Elger G, Hoppe C, Falkai, P, et al. (2000) Vagus nerve stimulation is associated with mood improvements in epilepsy patients. Epilepsy Res 42: 203–210.

Chapter 9
Resective Surgery for Patients with Epilepsy and Intellectual Disabilities

A. Nicolson

Introduction

Epilepsy is common in patients with intellectual disabilities (ID), and is often refractory to medical treatment. In one long-term study 70% of patients with an intelligence quoitent (IQ) less than 70 continued to have more than one seizure per year, compared to only 25% of those with borderline (IQ 71-85) or average (IQ >85) intelligence.[1] Such patients are therefore among those whose potentially could benefit most from epilepsy surgery.

When considering the possibility of epilepsy surgery one needs to consider the risks to the patient of ongoing refractory epilepsy. There is the ongoing risk of injury during seizures, and patients with ID and refractory epilepsy are among the highest at risk of sudden death (SUDEP).[2] Added to this are the major psychosocial and cognitive impacts that refractory epilepsy has upon the individual, and so surgical treatment deserves serious consideration in this population. Of course there will be individuals who have clear multiple seizure foci or symptomatic generalized epilepsy who will not be candidates for resective surgery, but many patients with ID and epilepsy may have surgically treatable lesions.

However, it has been a traditionally held view that a low IQ is a relative contraindication to surgery,[3–5] as the ID may represent a global brain dysfunction, with multiple seizure foci. Also of concern in patients with ID is the risk to cognitive functioning in patients with an already limited cognitive reserve. However, until recently this widely held belief has gone unchallenged, and as a consequence there are likely to be many patients who may benefit from surgery who are denied the appropriate evaluation. This is particularly crucial in children with ID and epilepsy whose global development will be adversely affected by ongoing seizure activity, and who may have the most to gain from early assessment for resective surgery.

V.P. Prasher, M.P. Kerr (eds.) *Epilepsy and Intellectual Disabilities*,
DOI: 10.1007/978-1-84800-259-3_9, © Springer Science+Business Media, LLC 2008

Should a Low IQ Be a Contraindication to Epilepsy Surgery?

The first major multicenter study to examine this issue analyzed data retrospectively from over 1,000 adults who had undergone temporal lobe resective surgery in eight centers in the United States[6] and had full pre- and postoperative neuropsychological assessments. Only 24 patients (2.3%) had an IQ less than 70, highlighting the tendency for such patients to not receive resective surgical treatment. This study did show a relationship between preoperative IQ and seizure outcome, but the effect was modest. Indeed the remission rate in those with an IQ less than 70 was 54.2%, and was 73.2% for those with a borderline IQ level. This emphasizes that although a lower IQ may predict a slightly worse outcome in some, there are a significant proportion of patients who can derive great benefit. The poorest outcome in this study was in those with a low IQ who had a structural lesion other than hippocampal sclerosis.

Several other small studies have also addressed this issue of preoperative IQ level and outcome following surgery. In 16 adults with an IQ less than 85, Gleissner and colleagues[7] found a remission rate of 64%, with no deterioration in neuropsychological function and some positive socioeconomic outcomes. The main predictor of a poor outcome was a left-sided lesion, which is likely to be because the surgery in the dominant hemisphere was more restricted.

The same group examined 285 consecutive children who underwent resective epilepsy surgery, and examined the outcome in relation to IQ level.[8] Twenty-one patients (7.4%) had an IQ less than 70, with 24 (8.4%) of below average level (IQ 71-85). There was no significant difference between these groups and those with an average IQ in terms of seizure outcome one year after surgery, with 67% seizure free in the low IQ group, 77% of those with a borderline IQ, and 78% in the group with average intelligence. No change was found in neuropsychological testing, other than an improvement in executive functioning of those with a low IQ. Attention improved and behavioral problems were less marked postoperatively in all groups.

Bjornaes and colleagues[9] found a remission rate of 48% in 31 patients with an IQ less than 70 who underwent resective surgery. Remission was more likely in those with temporal compared with extratemporal epilepsy (52% versus 38%), but the main factor predictive of outcome was the duration of epilepsy. In those with epilepsy for less than 12 years, 80% were seizure free. This raises the crucial issue of timing of epilepsy surgery in general, but in particular in this group with ID. It is well known that chronic refractory epilepsy has a negative neuropsychological and psychosocial effect, and it may be that rather than excluding patients with ID from the option of curative treatment, we should be more aggressive at an earlier stage.

There is a significantly higher rate of psychiatric problems in patients with epilepsy than the general population, particularly in those with drug-refractory partial epilepsy. A mood disorder is very common in such patients, and depending on the definition used, may occur in up to 75% of patients[10]; anxiety has been reported in over 40%[11] of individuals with refractory epilepsy. Suicide rates may be up to 25 times more common in patients with temporal lobe epilepsy compared with people without epilepsy.[12] It has been recognized that psychiatric symptoms may worsen or appear de novo following epilepsy surgery, and so surgery is often undertaken with extreme caution or refused on the grounds of pre-existing psychiatric problems. This issue may be of particular relevance to the ID population with epilepsy where behavioral problems and other psychiatric symptoms may coexist. Many clinicians may have reservations about epilepsy surgery in a patient with ID for the reasons already stated, and if they have psychiatric symptoms in addition, the patient is often rejected for surgery.

However, some reports have suggested that the psychiatric status of epilepsy patients is either not influenced, or may even improve, following epilepsy surgery[13,14] and that even patients with chronic psychosis may have a successful outcome.[15] The evidence for the psychiatric outcome in patients with ID is limited, but one of the studies examining the seizure outcome in patients with different IQ scores commented on an overall improvement in behavioral problems in patients with ID.[8]

A study of 226 consecutive patients who underwent epilepsy surgery at a single center showed a favorable psychiatric outcome overall[16] but did not specifically examine patients with ID. There was a high proportion (34.5%) of some psychiatric disturbance preoperatively, with psychosis in 16%. In 22 patients (28%) the psychiatric symptoms resolved post surgery; the main symptom was postictal psychosis, which suggests that this may be a factor favoring surgery. Thirty-nine patients (50%) had a persistence of psychiatric symptoms postoperatively, and the symptoms appeared de novo in 17 (22%). In many of those patients with new-onset psychiatric symptoms there were detectable personality traits presurgery that would predispose to psychiatric problems, which has been reported previously.[17] De novo postsurgery psychosis has been reported to be more common in nondominant resections[18,19] and some tumors such as gangliogliomas,[20] but this has not been confirmed in other studies.[16] Major depressive episodes may occur following epilepsy surgery, but these are usually transitory and in individuals with a history of a milder mood disorder.[17]

Despite concerns over performing surgery in patients with ID, recent evidence, albeit from small studies, suggests that a low IQ should not itself be an exclusion factor for resective epilepsy surgery. There may be a trend for patients who have more severe ID to have a slightly worse outcome, but still a significant proportion derive great benefit, with no evidence of worsening cognitive performance or behavior. However, further studies on this issue are required in larger numbers to confirm these findings and also to examine whether patients with a more severe ID may also benefit from resective surgery, as the data for the group with an IQ less than 50 are very limited. It seems intuitive that if surgery is to be considered, it should be undertaken as early as possible, rather than waiting for years of chronic drug-refractory epilepsy and the consequential negative impact that this has, particularly on a child's development. This will require a fundamental shift in thinking outside of specialist centers, as currently many such patients may be managed in the community or by psychiatrists with an interest in ID and may never have access to neurological and specialist epilepsy services.

Special Consideration for Presurgical Evaluation in People with LD

The main role of epilepsy surgery is to achieve seizure freedom, or a significant reduction in seizure frequency, without producing adverse cognitive or psychological effects. It has been proposed that epilepsy surgery should be considered in anyone "in whom the seizure represents the sole or predominant factor preventing a normal quality of life."[21] This may not be the case in individuals with ID, as achieving a "normal" quality of life may not be possible, and the goals of epilepsy surgery need to be carefully considered.

The investigative process in patients with ID may be even more complicated than in those with normal intelligence. Vital to accurate seizure localization is the correlation between clinical features, imaging, and electroencephalograms (EEG). Patients with ID may not be as able as those with a higher IQ to give a detailed account of their seizure symptomatology, magnetic resonance imaging (MRI) may be difficult without a general anesthetic, and neuropsychological testing needs to take the low IQ into account.

Neuropsychological Assessment

There are several aims of the preoperative neuropsychological assessment in all patients in an epilepsy surgery program. It gives us information about the cerebral organization of an individual's verbal and visuospatial skills and determines any evidence for areas of brain dysfunction which could be relevant to the seizure focus. It also examines the postoperative risk to memory and language skills. An essential part of the assessment, in addition to these principal functions, is to evaluate the potential psychosocial consequences of surgery to that individual. This includes the identification of any psychiatric comorbidity and the evaluation of the patient's (and family's or caregiver's) expectations about surgery. How a patient copes with epilepsy and his or her preoperative support network are relevant when identifying the possible psychosocial consequences of successful surgery. Patients are more likely to perceive the surgery as a success if their goals have been realistic and practical before surgery.[22] The change from having frequent seizures that negatively impact social lives, employment, driving, and relationships to being seizure free after surgery is a major life event that can be difficult to adjust to.[23] The goals from surgery for patients with ID may vary considerably from those without such a disability. However, this may be difficult to ascertain easily, and specific counseling about this issue is essential for the patient and family or caregivers.

These factors are applicable to any candidates for epilepsy surgery, but special consideration may be required for individuals with ID. The neuropsychological assessment tools are not specific to individuals with ID, and it is not known whether they provide as accurate a picture of overall cognitive functioning as in people with average intelligence. The actual neuropsychological tests used vary widely between centers — there is no uniform approach,[24] and there is no specific protocol for patients with ID. This is also particularly relevant to children with ID, who provide their own unique challenges. It is likely that at different ages during childhood certain neuropsychological methods may be most beneficial or alternatively difficult to interpret.

The intracarotid amytal, or Wada, test is established as a method of examining laterality of language functioning and predicting those at risk of postoperative amnesia. As with standard neuropsychological testing, the procedure varies between centers, and some feel it is not a necessary investigation when baseline neuropsychometry provides clear evidence for lateralization.[25] When the test is performed, the sodium amytal is injected into a single carotid artery to provide anesthesia of one hemisphere, enabling the neuropsychologist to test the memory and language abilities of the contralateral hemisisphere. Whether the Wada test is valid, or requires modification, in patients with ID is not known, and some do not perform this test in individuals with an IQ below 75.[24] It may be that in the future other methods will replace the role of the Wada test, in particular functional MRI (fMRI) (Figure 9.1AD) and magnetoencephalography (MEG), but any protocols developed in these technologies may need to be adapted for people with ID.

Seizure Recordings

Seizure recordings are routinely required in the presurgical evaluation process, and even in the most clear-cut cases it is valuable in confirming seizure semiology. In patients with ID, obtaining seizure recordings may be more problematic, and measures such as allowing caregivers to stay with the patient may be required. Reducing medication on the day of admission may help to shorten the length of hospital stay. Often in cases associated with ID the seizure focus cannot be reliably determined with scalp EEG recordings and routine MRI, and so invasive depth or subdural strips/grids are required (Figure 9.2). Such procedures may be more difficult for patients with ID to tolerate, and if any intraoperative mapping is required, this may be very difficult.

Consent

At every stage during the presurgical evaluation process it is essential that every effort is made to ensure that informed consent is given. This may be difficult in patients with ID, and although in this situation a legal guardian will have to provide assent it is of paramount importance that professionals experienced in dealing with such patients and their families undergo detailed discussions about the aims, risks, and expectations from investigations or procedures.

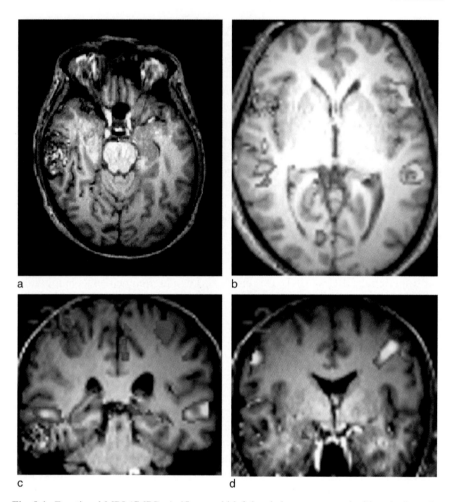

Fig. 9.1 Functional MRI (fMRI). A 45-year-old left-handed man presented with a single tonic-clonic seizure; MRI revealed a right temporal lobe arteriovenous malformation (AVM) (A). During the evaluation process for surgical excision of the AVM he underwent fMRI for language localization. This was carried out with three different language paradigms. The verb generation paradigm demonstrated bilateral Broca's and Wernicke area activation, with the Wernicke's area just superior to the nidus of the AVM on the right (B-D)

Pathologies Associated with ID That May Benefit from Resective Surgery

Focal Cortical Dysplasia

Focal cortical dysplasia (FCD) was first described over 30 years ago,[26] and while our abilities to detect it have improved significantly with new imaging techniques, uncertainties about FCD remain.

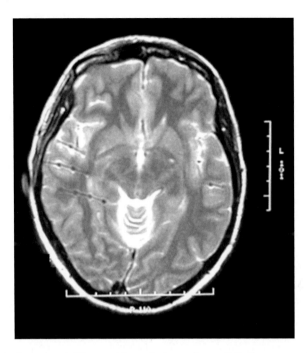

Fig. 9.2 Depth electrodes. A 25-year-old man had complex partial seizures preceded by a stereotyped olfactory aura. MRI was normal, and ictal scalp EEG recordings had suggested that the seizures had a right temporal onset. This was confirmed with depth electrode recordings, with three electrodes placed in the right temporal lobe and one in the left temporal lobe

Focal cortical dysplasia is commonly associated with severe drug-resistant epilepsy, including epilepsia partialis continua; therefore, evaluation for potential surgery is increasingly important. Focal cortical dysplasia is frequently associated with a degree of ID, and many cases that were previously termed cryptogenic may now have FCD identified with high-resolution MRI, although even the most sophisticated MRI will not currently identify all cases of FCD and therefore the true prevalence of FCD is not known. Surgery offers some hope to patients with FCD, as antiepileptic drugs (AEDs) will often fail to achieve remission.

Several surgical series have been published on the outcome of patients undergoing surgery for FCD, with reported remission rates mostly around 40–50%[27–34] but with some studies showing rates as high as 70–90%.[35–40] As with any reports of data from surgical series one needs to take into account different methodologies when interpreting the data, such as patient numbers, selection criteria, and length of follow-up in particular. We know from studies of surgical outcome in patients with hippocampal sclerosis that late relapses can occur,[41] and a lengthy follow-up is needed to accurately predict prognosis. One such study reported a 10-year follow-up of patients who underwent surgery for malformations of cortical development (MCD), 31 of whom had FCD.[30] In the group overall, the remission rate remained stable between 2 years and 10 years, suggesting that patients with MCD who initially do well following epilepsy surgery are likely to have a favorable long-term outcome. However, in another

study of 49 patients with FCD the proportion of patients with a favorable postoperative seizure outcome following surgery dropped from 84% to 70% over the 10 years
of follow-up, and most of this change was observed during the first 3 years.[34]

Several studies have identified factors that may predict outcome from surgery,
with completeness of resection commonly identified.[30,33,42] As with other pathologies,
outcome has also been dependent on the location of the lesion, with extratemporal
FCD having a poorer surgical outcome.[29,43] Attempts have been made to examine
whether the histological subtype of FCD influences outcome, with varying results.
Cortical dysplasia can be classified in order of cytological disruption as "mild malformation of cortical development" (mMCD) or FCD type 1a (isolated architectural
abnormalities); 1b (with additional immature or giant neurons); 2a (with additional
dysmorphic neurons); and 2b (with additional balloon cells) (Figure 9.3).[44]
This is a pathological classification system, and we do not currently know how this
correlates with clinical features and severity of the epilepsy or outcome following surgery.
It is clear, however, that the patients with FCD are a heterogenous group. One study

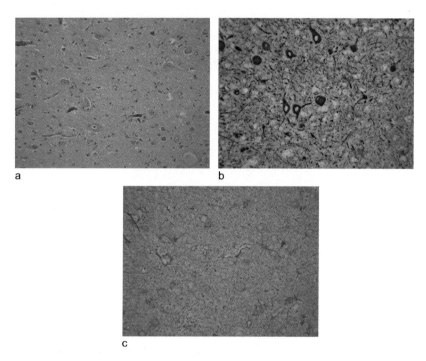

a   b

c

Fig. 9.3 Histological slide of focal cortical dysplasia. Photomicrograph depicting an abnormal
cluster of dysplastic neurons with irregular profiles closely admixed with large, binucleated astro-
glial cells exhibiting pale pink cytoplasm (A). When stained with neurofilament protein this shows
the perikaryion of the neurons and their axons embedded in a disorganised neuropil background
(B). On the slide stained with GFAP (Glial Fibrillary Acidic Protein) stroglial cells are highlighted
in close apposition to the neurons (which remain unstained) (C). A subpopulation of cells exhibiting co-localisation of reactivity with both Neurofilament protein and GFAP, suggestive of a
dysplastic nature of divergent phenotype

that examined whether the histological subtype of FCD influenced surgical outcome found a trend towards better results in those patients with a less severe histological subtype (mMCD or FCD type 1a),[32] but this study has relatively small numbers with limited follow-up. Others have found the reverse situation, with outcome better in FCD 2[39] or no correlation.[34] This issue clearly needs evaluation in larger studies with longer follow-up data, which would allow us to further our understanding of the clinicopathological correlate in FCD and ultimately enable us to identify presurgery those candidates who are likely to have the most favorable outcome. With a condition such as FCD, this will only be possible with multicenter collaboration.

Focal cortical dysplasia can coexist as "dual pathology" with other pathologies which are also known to cause epilepsy, such as hippocampal sclerosis (HS) and dysembryoplastic neuroepithelial tumors (DNT). Certain dual pathologies have an unfavorable outcome following epilepsy surgery, for example HS with periventricular nodular heterotopia,[45] but some small studies suggest that if both pathologies are readily identifiable presurgery and considered resectable then the outcome is favorable. A study of 28 patients with temporal lobe epilepsy associated with FCD found no difference in the outcome between those patients with FCD only and those with additional HS.[35] In a study of patients with DNT who underwent surgical resection, an associated cortical dysplasia was identified in over 80% of patients.[46] This finding emphasizes that in tumors such as DNT a focal resection may not be sufficient to achieve remission, and in many the surrounding tissue may be dysplastic and "epileptogenic." Other authors have also reported that in cases of temporal lobe dual pathology the outcome is good if the lesions are resected in addition to the mesial temporal structures.[47,48]

In the past decade the identification of FCD has been revolutionized by advances in MRI techniques in particular, but still this may not identify FCD in up to 30% of patients.[49] Characteristic findings on MRI are an abnormal gyral pattern, increased cortical thickness, poor grey-white matter differentiation, and increased subcortical signal on T2-weighted and FLAIR images.[50] Detailed presurgical evaluation is necessary to identify the epileptogenic zone, and this is a particular challenge in those patients with normal MRIs. As imaging techniques improve, it seems likely that more patients with FCD will be able to be identified and become surgical candidates. Currently, as a routine in the presurgical evaluation process these patients should undergo high-resolution MRI and scalp video-EEG telemetry. In some patients this will be sufficient to identify the FCD, but in others techniques such as intracranial EEG recordings, positron emission tomography (PET), or ictal single-photon emission computed tomography (SPECT)[51] will be required. Ictal SPECT identifies the epileptogenic zone as a an area of hyperperfusion based on cerebral metabolic and perfusion coupling,[52] and an early injection can reduce the risk of identifying a postictal hypoperfused area. SPECT coregistered to MRI (SISCOM) (Figure 9.4) may identify a localized region of cerebral perfusion concordant with the epileptogenic zone[53] and improve the localizing value of ictal SPECT. Patients are most likely to have a favorable seizure outcome if the focal cortical resection includes the region of peri-ictal blood flow change.[53,54] Ictal SPECT and SISCOM may be particularly useful in patients with FCD which is not identifiable on standard MR imaging.

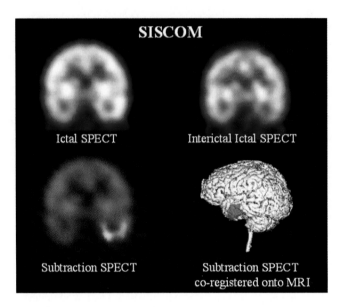

Fig. 9.4 Ictal SPECT coregistered to MRI (SISCOM). SISCOM in a patient with right temporal lobe epilepsy. Routine MRI was normal. Note that the right side of the brain is on the right side of the figure

Our knowledge of FCD has advanced significantly in recent years, but the major challenges of being able to identify all patients with FCD preoperatively and to verify whether there are subgroups of patients who are most likely to respond well to surgery remain.

Other Malformations of Cortical Development

Schizencephaly is a malformation of cortical development (MCD) that consists of congenital clefts in the cerebral mantle extending from the pial surface to the lateral ventricles and lined by cortical gray matter.[55] It may have a variable clinical presentation ranging from little or no deficit to severe developmental delay, hemiplegia, and epilepsy, which often will be refractory to AED treatment. The structural changes may be unilateral or bilateral, and when unilateral surgery may be considered. However, data on the outcome of surgery in patients with schizencephaly are limited,[56–58] and the evaluation process is likely to be complex. Even when the cleft is unilateral it may be multilobar, the structural abnormality may be distant from the epileptogenic zone, and the dysplastic cortex may be essential for language and motor functions.[59] Invasive EEG recordings are required in such patients, but SISCOM may provide useful data to guide electrode placement and/or cortical resection.[60] In the reported cases the surgical strategy has varied and includes temporal lobectomy, excision of the dysplastic cortex, and resection of cortex distant from the cleft. Polymicrogyria is an MCD characterized by an increase in the number and decrease in the size of gyri; it may be generalized or localized. It has a widely varying clinical presentation which depends upon the distribution of the dysplastic cortex and the presence of any other underlying abnormality. In some patients with refractory epilepsy a focal potentially resectable region may be identifiable.[61]

MRI has improved our recognition of uncommon MCDs such as schizencephaly and polymicrogyria. The majority of these patients are managed medically, but surgery may be an option for some with unilateral dysplastic cortex.

Dysembryoplastic Neuroepithelial Tumor (DNT)

Dysembryoplastic neuroepithelial tumors are benign glioneuronal tumors frequently associated with refractory epilepsy in children and young adults.[62] They have characteristic findings on imaging with a mixed signal lesion on MRI which is based in the cortex but may involve the white matter, often with overlying skull abnormalities indicating a chronic lesion.[63] They typically have a disorganized arrangement of neuronal and glial elements without cytological atypia and frequent association of foci of dysplastic cortical disorganization. Cortical dysplasia is frequently associated with DNTs,[63–71] which need careful evaluation preoperatively, as a high proportion of associated "MRI-invisible" cortical dysplasia has been reported.[46] For optimum surgical outcome, this needs to be identified presurgically by invasive methods (intracranial EEG recordings and/or electrocorticography) to ensure resection of the entire epileptogenic zone,[72,73] but in some patients functional imaging such as SISCOM may provide a noninvasive alternative.[74]

Intellectual disability may occur in around 40% of cases with DNT,[75] but the presence of LD may imply a more widespread cortical dysfunction. DNTs are often surgically resectable, with studies generally showing a favorable outcome in terms of seizure control,[62,63,66,67,76–80] but the outcome is less certain in patients with ID.

Tuberous Sclerosis

Tuberous sclerosis complex (TSC) is an autosomal dominant neurocutaneous syndrome with variable expression and a high spontaneous mutation rate, which is characterized by multiple hamartomas in the skin, retina, heart, kidney, and brain. It is associated with epilepsy in up to 90% of cases, which is usually of early onset and refractory to medical treatment in up to 30%.[81] The central nervous system involvement in TSC also gives rise to focal neurological deficits and developmental and intellectual delay. There is evidence that achieving early seizure control may have a positive impact on cognitive development and social adjustment.[82] Traditionally, epilepsy surgery has not been considered an option for TSC patients, as imaging often reveals multiple tubers and therefore potentially multiple epileptogenic zones.

However, in certain cases surgery may be a realistic option, particularly for those patients with stereotyped seizures that suggest an origin from a single tuber.

The presurgical assessment of a patient with TSC offers some unique challenges. Magnetic resonance imaging will often reveal multiple tubers in TSC and does not identify the origin of the seizures,[83] and interictal EEG may show multiple abnormalities or be nonlocalizing.[84–86] On MRI, FLAIR sequences, or even diffusion-weighted imaging,[87] may be optimal to detect tubers. Computerized tomography can be useful to identify calcification, one study suggesting that such tubers may be more likely to be epileptogenic.[88] In some cases with TSC the epileptogenic tuber will be relatively easy to identify with concordance between MRI, interictal, and ictal EEG. However, in many cases invasive EEG recordings with depth electrodes and/or subdural grids will be necessary. Functional imaging such as ictal SPECT can aid localization with hyperperfusion anterior to the epileptogenic tuber.[89] FDG-PET scans may reveal multiple hypometabolic regions corresponding anatomically to the tubers, and will not differentiate between those with or without epileptogenic potential.[90–92] Other radioactive ligands such as C-alpha-methyl-tryptophan (CAMT), a marker of serotonin synthesis, may be more promising in this regard, as this has been shown to have a significantly greater uptake in epileptogenic tubers.[93,94] FDG-PET coregistration with MRI and diffusion tensor imaging may provide additional information to PET alone.[95]

At present, such functional imaging techniques, and more recently SISCOM, are useful tools to aid localization, but in practice invasive EEG recordings are usually required and this information can assist with the placement of such electrodes. Invasive monitoring can also identify adjacent functional cortex to guide resection. MEG is a technique that selectively measures tangential sources (e.g., sources on a sulcus) rather than the radial sources also detected by EEG. MEG can be combined with EEG recordings simultaneously and then visualized by plotting the equivalent current dipole on the patient's MRI brain scan with volume reconstruction.

Experience in localizing the epileptogenic zone with MEG is limited in TSC, but some provisional studies have suggested that it may have a role,[96,97] and in combination with PET and ictal SPECT could provide a three-dimensional map of the relation of the epileptic activity to the adjacent structural and functional anatomy.

Several small series of cases of surgically treated TSC have been reported, with a remission rate between 10% and 78% (Table 9.1).

The best outcome is for:

1. Patients with a single seizure type or single tuber
2. Patients with multiple tubers and one large calcified tuber, with concordant interictal EEG abnormalities related to it
3. Patients with concordant investigationsAlthough the evaluation process is more complicated and potentially higher risk, patients who do not fall into these good prognostic groups should not be denied appropriate investigation. There are reports of successful outcomes in cases requiring multistage investigation and surgery, even for bilateral seizure foci.[111,112]

The multifocal nature of TSC means that when undergoing resective surgery special consideration needs to be given to the possibility of further epileptogenic

Table 9.1 Selected series of resective surgery for tuberous sclerosis patients (modified from Romanelli and colleagues.[98]

Author	No. of Patients	Remission Rate (%)	Follow-up (months)
Bebin[99]	9	67	38
Avellino[100]	8	55	35
Baumgartner[101]	4	0	30
Guerreiro[102]	12	58	120
Acharya[103]	9	78	1 mon-14 yrs
Neville[104]	6	67	60
Koh[88]	13	69	48
Thiele[105]	21	33	50
Karenfort[106]	8	38	42
Vigliano[107]	4	75	24
Sinclair[108]	4	78	60
Jarrar[109]	21	42	60
Lachhwani[110]	17	65	25

tubers developing, and patients need to be counseled accordingly. One study found that in this patient group the remission rate fell from 59% (13 of 21) to 42% after five years,[109] but larger systematic long-term studies are required to see whether this phenomenon is more common in TSC patients than others with a different underlying pathology such as FCD or hippocampal sclerosis.

Lennox-Gastaut Syndrome

Lennox-Gastaut syndrome (LGS) is a form of symptomatic generalized epilepsy that is characterized by a peak age of onset between two and six years of age, multiple seizure types, a characteristic EEG abnormality, and often severe ID. Approximately one third of children will have had West syndrome in the first year of life. Symptomatic cases may be caused by focal, multifocal, or diffuse cerebral abnormalities, which could be congenital or acquired.

As LGS is a generalized epilepsy syndrome, it typically is not amenable to resective surgery. However, atypical LGS may be related to a focal lesion, and if such a lesion is identified on MRI, it may be possible to identify a resectable epileptogenic zone and provide a good seizure outcome.[113,114]

Hemispherectomy

The technique of hemispherectomy was first used to treat refractory epilepsy in Toronto in 1938.[115] After the technique was utilized in a number of cases,[116] it became apparent that there was a significant associated mortality and morbidity, and in particular a high risk of the development of superficial siderosis, due to hemorrhage into the fluid-filled cavity left by the removal of the hemisphere. The hemispherectomy only became an accepted treatment for refractory epilepsy caused by diffuse hemispheric syndromes when the technique was modified by Rasmussen.[117,118]

Hemispherectomy is indicated as a treatment for refractory partial seizures secondary to a diffuse hemispheric abnormality. Presurgical evaluation is required to ensure that seizures originate solely from the affected hemisphere, and that the contralateral hemisphere is normal. Magnetic resonance imaging can determine whether there is any structural abnormality, and functional techniques such as PET, SPECT (showing interictal hypoperfusion and ictal hyperperfusion from the affected hemisphere), fMRI, and MEG can evaluate the functions of the hemispheres in terms of motor, sensory, and language functions. Further localization may be performed with intracranial recordings with subdural strips or grids, which provide intraoperative mapping of eloquent cortex.

The ideal timing for hemispherectomy is uncertain. Earlier intervention will reduce the adverse cognitive effects of years of poorly controlled seizures and the sedative effects of AEDs and subsequently improve quality of life. However, it is uncertain whether surgical intervention should be delayed until neurological deficits such as hemiparesis or dysphasia become established, or to perform the procedure as early as possible. Although there is evidence for a better cognitive outcome in cases of Sturge-Weber syndrome (SWS) if hemispherectomy is performed during the first year of life,[119] there is also fMRI evidence that sensory and motor functions may transfer to the contralateral hemisphere at different stages of cerebral maturation[120] and that postponement of surgery until completion of transfer of functions from the diseased to intact hemisphere leads to better fine and motor function.[121] A fine balance clearly is required to consider both of these factors in each individual being considered for hemispherectomy.

One of the major indications for hemispherectomy is Sturge-Weber syndrome (SWS) (Figure 9.5), a neurocutaneous syndrome characterized by a facial capillary angioma (port-wine stain) seen predominantly in the distribution of the first branch of the trigeminal nerve; however, it may be more extensive, with an underlying leptomeningeal angioma that can occasionally be bilateral. The leptomenigeal angioma may be detected by skull X-ray, CT, or MRI. Typically SWS is associated with a moderate to severe ID (a normal IQ occurs in only 25-30%)[122] and refractory epilepsy. Status epilepticus is common, and there may be periods of encephalopathy associated with cognitive and developmental plateau and increased hemiplegia.[123] Although the leptomeningeal angioma may be easily evident on standard imaging, the epileptogenic zone may be more extensive; seizure recordings thus are essential, and intraoperative electrocorticography may be used to guide the extent of resection.[124]

Any other conditions that cause a diffuse unilateral hemispheric disorder and epilepsy may be considered for hemispherectomy, in particular hemimegalencephaly (a neuronal migration disorder resulting in a unilateral enlarged hemisphere), Rasmussen's encephalitis, hemiconvulsion-hemiplegia, and epilepsy (HHE) syndrome, and a spastic hemiplegia caused by perinatal stroke.

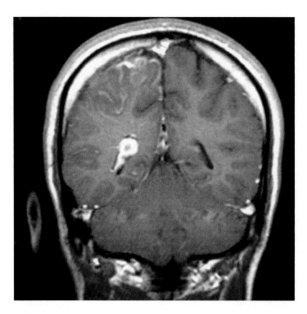

Fig. 9.5 Sturge-Weber syndrome. Post-contrast MRI shows the characteristic features of Sturge-Weber syndrome with abnormal enhancement, suggesting calcification in the cortical veins, together with right hemisphere atrophy

Several small series of the outcome from hemispherectomy have been reported, with generally favorable results. One of the largest series with prolonged follow-up found that 65% of 111 children who underwent hemispherectomy were seizure free, and 89% could walk without assistance. The poorest seizure outcome was found in those with neuronal migration disorders.[125] Another study of 115 patients found the poorest outcome and most complicated surgery in cases of hemimegalencephaly, but not in those with unilateral hemisphere cortical dysplasia, i.e., without the abnormally enlarged hemisphere.[126] Other series have produced remission rates of 52–81%[127–132] with a generally good motor outcome, usually cognitive stability or improvement, and behavioral improvement in many.

Since the earlier anatomical hemispherectomy technique was found to be associated with an unacceptable degree of complications, the technique has evolved to more restricted resections with disconnections. The functional hemispherectomy was first described in 1983 and entails the resection of the parietal and temporal lobes, Rolandic region, and severing the connections with the thalamus and brainstem, hence leaving in place the frontal and occipital lobes and their blood supply. This procedure has a much lower risk of the complication of hemosiderosis (in a series of 20 patients none had hemosiderosis[133]) compared with up to 30% of patients undergoing anatomical hemispherectomy,[134] although it should be stressed that some series of patients undergoing anatomical hemispherectomy also report no cases of haemosiderosis.[135] The disadvantage of the functional hemispherectomy is that the potentially epileptogenic insula is left in situ, although the seizure freedom

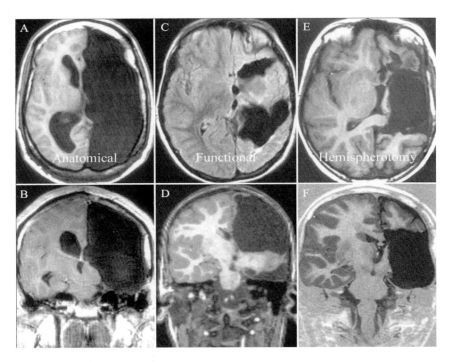

Fig. 9.6 Hemispherectomy. T1-Weighted MRI scans of examples of anatomical (A and B) and functional (C and D) hemispherectomy, and hemispherotomy (E and F)

rates compare favorably with the conventional procedure.[136] Other more restricted procedures include hemicorticectomy (only grey matter is resected) and hemispherotomy (disconnection of the epileptogenic hemisphere from the subcortical centers, thereby reducing brain excision (See Figure 9.6)).

Patients with the diffuse hemispheric disorders discussed here often have severe epilepsy with profound developmental and cognitive delay and hemiplegia. In childhood this is the patient group with potentially the most to gain from successful epilepsy surgery, as this can provide dramatic benefits not only in terms of seizure control but particularly cognitive development, and further work needs to be done to enable us to make an appropriate judgement on the timing of surgery.

Evaluating the Outcome of Resective Epilepsy Surgery in Patients with ID

The immediate aim of resective epilepsy surgery is to reduce, and hopefully stop, seizures. However, there are many other additional factors that are vitally important in assessing the overall outcome in terms of quality of life. The ultimate aim has to be to improve quality of life, which is not achieved if the patient has fewer seizures but an adverse cognitive or psychiatric outcome. Even seizure freedom does not necessarily improve quality of life, and many such patients may continue to lead a "disabled" life with no discernable functional benefit.[34, 137]

An essential part of the presurgical evaluation is to assess the patient's and/or caregiver's expectations of surgery, and careful counseling at this point may ensure that these are not unrealistically high. This is particularly relevant in patients with ID in whom even the most favorable seizure outcome may not lead to as much of an improvement in functioning as caregivers may hope for or expect. However, the possibility of a reduction of seizure frequency and severity and a reduction in the drug burden are valid reasons to consider epilepsy surgery in this patient group, which may have particularly severe and frequent seizures, and so be in a particularly high-risk group for seizure-related injury and death (SUDEP).

There is not an established health-related quality of life measure that reliably assesses the impact that epilepsy surgery has on the quality of life of an individual with ID or their family. To measure this is complex and requires the evaluation of multiple domains and so requires the use of a variety of instruments of quality of life.

Conclusion

The traditionally held view that patients with ID will not be candidates for consideration of epilepsy surgery has been challenged in recent years. No longer are palliative procedures such as corpus callosotomy the only surgical options in such cases, and prospects of seizure freedom are realistic for many with ID. It would seem that a subgroup of patients with focal epilepsy and ID can be identified and treated successfully without drastic cognitive consequences. However, resective epilepsy surgery in the ID population remains a significant challenge. The identification of suitable candidates may be difficult, and the evaluation procedure may require special considerations and adaptations for those with ID. Newer techniques such as higher-resolution MRI have aided us in identifying potentially resectable epileptogenic foci, and in the future advances in technologies such as fMRI, SISCOM, and MEG may help further to localize foci more accurately and noninvasively, which would carry benefits for all patients with refractory focal epilepsy, including those with ID.

References

1. Huttenlocher PR, Hapke RJ. (1990) A follow-up study of intractable seizures in childhood. Ann Neurol 28:699–705.
2. Nashef L, Fish DR, Allen P et al. (1995) Incidence of sudden unexpected death in an adult outpatient cohort with epilepsy at a tertiary referral centre. J Neurol Neurosurg Psychiatr 58: 462–4.
3. Falconer MA.(1973) Reversibility by temporal lobe resection of the behavioural abnormalities of temporal-lobe epilepsy. N Engl J Med 289: 451–5.

4. Rasmussen T. (1975) Surgical treatment of patients with complex partial seizures. Adv Neurol 11:415–49.
5. Engel J, Jr. Surgery for seizures. (1996) N Engl J Med 334:647–52.
6. Chelune GJ, Naugle RI, Hermann BP, et al. (1998) Does presurgical IQ predict seizure outcome after temporal lobectomy? Evidence from the Bozeman epilepsy consortium. Epilepsia 39:314–8.
7. Gleissner U, Johanson K, Helmstaedter C, et al. (1999) Surgical outcome in a group of low-IQ patients with focal epilepsy. Epilepsia. 40: 553–9.
8. Gleissner U, Clusmann H, Sassen R, et al. (2006) Postsurgical outcome in pediatric patients with epilepsy: A comparison of patients with intellectual disabilities, subaverage intelligence, and average-range intelligence. Epilepsia. 47: 406–14.
9. Bjornaes H, Stabell KE, Heminghyt E, et al. (2004) Resective surgery for intractable focal epilepsy in patients with low IQ: Predictors for seizure control and outcome with respect to seizures and neuropsychological and psychosocial functioning. Epilepsia. 45: 131–9.
10. Indaco A, Carrieri PB, Nappi C, et al. (1992) Interictal depression in epilepsy. Epilepsy Res 12: 45–50.
11. Bladin PF. (1992) Psychosocial difficulties and outcome after temporal lobectomy. Epilepsia 33: 898–907.
12. Barraclough B. (1981) Suicide and epilepsy. In: Reynolds EH, Trimble MR (eds.). Epilepsy and psychiatry. Edinburgh: Churchill Livingstone, 72–6.
13. Fenwick P. (1991) Long-term psychiatric outcome after epilepsy surgery. In: Luders HO (ed.). Epilepsy surgery. New York: Raven Press, 647–52.
14. Savard G, Andermann F, Olivier A, et al. (1991) Postictal psychosis after partial complex seizures: A multiple case study. Epilepsia 32: 225–31.
15. Reutens Dc, Savard G, Andermann F, et al. (1997) Results of surgical treatment in temporal lobe epilepsy with chronic psychosis. Brain 120: 1929–36.
16. Inoue Y, Mihara T. (2001) Psychiatric disorders before and after surgery for epilepsy. Epilepsia 42(Suppl 6): 13–18.
17. Koch-Stoecker S. (2001) Psychiatric outcome. In: Luders HO, Comair YG (eds.). Epilepsy surgery. Philadelphia: Lippincott Williams & Wilkins, 837–44.
18. Mace CJ, Trimble MR. (1991) Psychosis following temporal lobe surgery: A report of six cases. J Neurol Neurosurg Psychiatr 54: 639–44.
19. Trimble MR. (1992) Behaviour changes following temporal lobectomy, with special reference to psychosis. J Neurol Neurosurg Psychiatr 55: 89–91.
20. Bruton CJ. (1988) The neuropathology of temporal lobe epilepsy (Maudsley Monographs 31). Oxford: Oxford University Press.
21. Dreifuss FE. (1987) Goals of surgery for epilepsy. In: Engel J Jr (ed.). Surgical treatment of the epilepsies. New York: Raven Press, 31–49.
22. Wilson SJ, Saling MM, Kincade P, et al. (1998) Patient expectations of temporal lobe surgery. Epilepsia 39: 167–74.
23. Wheelock I, Peterson C, Buchtel HA. (1998) Presurgery expectations, postsurgery satisfaction, and psychosocial adjustment after epilepsy surgery. Epilepsia 639: 487–94.
24. Baker GA. (2001) Psychological and neuropsychological assessment before and after surgery for epilepsy: Implications for the management of learning-disabled people. Epilepsia 42(Suppl. 1): 41–3.
25. Baxendale S, Thompson P, Duncan J, et al. (2003) Is it time to replace the Wada test? Neurology 60: 354–5.
26. Taylor DC, Falconer MA, Bruton CI, et al. (1971) Focal dysplasia of the cerebral cortex in epilepsy. J Neurol Neurosurg Psychiatr 34: 369–87.
27. Sisodiya SM. (2000) Surgery for malformations of cortical development causing epilepsy. Brain 123: 1075–91.
28. Bast T, Ramantani G, Seitz A, et al. (2006) Focal cortical dysplasia: Prevalence, clinical presentation and epilepsy in children and adults. Acta Neurol Scand 113: 72–81.
29. Chung CK, Lee SK, Kim KJ. (2005) Surgical outcome of epilepsy caused by cortical dysplasia. Epilepsia 46(Suppl 1): 25–9.

30. Hamiwka L, Jayakar P, Resnick T, et al. (2005) Surgery for epilepsy due to cortical malformations: Ten-year follow-up. Epilepsia. 46: 556–60.
31. Siegel AM, Cascino GD, Meyer FB, et al. (2006) Surgical outcome and predictive factors in adult patients with intractable epilepsy and focal cortical dysplasia. Acta Neurol Scand 113:65–71.
32. Fauser S, Schulze-Bonhage A, Honegger J, et al. (2004) Focal cortical dysplasias: Surgical outcome in 67 patients in relation to histological subtypes and dual pathology. Brain 127: 2406–18.
33. Hader WJ, MacKay M, Otsubo H, et al. (2004) Cortical dysplastic lesions in children with intractable epilepsy: Role of complete resection. J Neurosurg (Pediatrics 2). 100: 110–7.
34. Srikijvilaikul T, Najm IM, Hovinga CA, et al. (2003) Seizure outcome after temporal lobectomy in temporal lobe cortical dysplasia. Epilepsia 44: 1420–4.
36. Hudgins RJ, Flamini JR, Palasis S, et al. (2005) Surgical treatment of epilepsy in children caused by focal cortical dysplasia. Pediatr Neurosurg 41: 70–6.
37. Cohen-Gadol AA, Ozduman K, Bronen RA, et al. (2004) Long-term outcome after epilepsy surgery for focal cortical dysplasia. J Neurosurg 101: 55–65.
38. Chassoux F, Devaux B, Landre E, et al. (2000) Stereoelectroencephalography in focal cortical dysplasia: A 3D approach to delineating the dysplastic cortex. Brain 123: 1733–51.
39. Tassi L, Colombo N, Garbelli R, et al. (2002) R. Focal cortical dysplasia: Neuropathological subtypes, EEG, neuroimaging and surgical outcome. Brain 125: 1719–32.
40. Kral T, Clusmann H, Blumcke I, et al. (2003) Outcome of epilepsy surgery in focal cortical dysplasia. J Neurol Neurosurg Psychiatr 74: 183–8.
41. McIntosh AM, Kalnins RM, Mitchell LA, et al. (2004) Temporal lobectomy: Long-term seizure outcome, late recurrence and risks for seizure recurrence. Brain 127: 2018–30.
42. Sisodiya SM. (2004) Surgery for focal cortical dysplasia. Brain 127: 2383–4.
43. Hirabayashi S, Binnie CD, Janota I, et al. (1993) Surgical treatment of epilepsy due to cortical dysplasia: Clinical and EEG findings. J Neurol Neurosurg Psychiatr 56: 765–70.
44. Palmini A, Najm I, Avanzini G. (2004) Terminology and classification of the cortical dysplasias. Neurology 62(Suppl 3): S2–8.
45. Li LM, Dubeau F, Andermann F, et al. (1997) Periventricular nodular hetrotopia and intractable temporal lobe epilepsy: Poor outcome after temporal lobe resection. Ann Neurol 41: 662–8.
46. Takahashi A, Hong S-C, Seo DW, et al. (2005) Frequent association of cortical dysplasia in dysembryoplastic neuroepithelial tumor treated by epilepsy surgery. Surg Neurol 64: 419–27.
47. Salanova V, Markand O, Worth R. (2004) Temporal lobe epilepsy: Analysis of patients with dual pathology. Acta Neurol Scand 109: 126–31.
48. Li LM, Cendes F, Andermann F, et al. (1999) Surgical outcome in patients with epilepsy and dual pathology. Brain 122:799–805.
49. Bautista JF, Foldvary-Schaefer N, Bingaman WE, et al. (2003) Focal cortical dysplasia and intractable epilepsy in adults: Clinical, EEG, imaging and surgical features. Epilepsy Res 55: 131–6.
50. Kuzniecky RI, Barkovich AJ. (2001) Malformations of cortical development and epilepsy. Brain Dev 23: 2–11.
51. Gupta A, Raja S, Kotagal P, et al. (2004) Ictal SPECT in children with partial epilepsy due to focal cortical dysplasia. Pediatr Neurol 131: 89–95.
52. Van Paesschen W. (2004) Ictal SPECT. Epilepsia 45(Suppl 4): 35–40.
53. O'Brien TJ, So EL, Mullan BP, et al. (1998) Subtraction ictal SPECT co-registered to MRI improves clinical usefulness of SPECT in localizing the surgical seizure focus. Neurology. 50: 445–54.
54. O'Brien TJ, So EL, Cascino GD, et al. (2004) Subtraction SPECT co-registered with MRI in focal malformations of cortical development: Localization of the epileptic zone in epilepsy surgery candidates. Epilepsia 45: 367–76.
55. Barkovich AJ, Normand D. (1988) MR imaging of schizencephaly. Am J Radiol 150: 1391–6.

56. Leblanc R, Tampieri D, Robitaille Y, et al. (1991) Surgical treatment of intractable epilepsy associated with schizencephaly. Neurosurgery 29: 421–9.
57. Landy HJ, Ramsey RE, Ajmoine-Marsan C, et al. (1992) Temporal lobectomy for seizures associated with unilateral schizencephaly. Surg Neurol 37: 477–81.
58. Silbergeld DL, Miller JW. (1994) Resective surgery for medically intractable epilepsy associated with schizencephaly. J Neurosurg 80: 820–5.
59. Jansky J, Ebner A, Kruse B, et al. (2003) Functional organization of the brain with malformations of cortical development. Ann Neurol 53: 759–67.
60. Cascino GD, Buchhalter JR, Sirven JI, et al. (2004) Peri-ictal SPECT and surgical treatment for intractable epilepsy related to schizencephaly. Neurology 63: 2426–8.
61. Cross JH, Jayakar P, Nordli D, et al. (2006) Proposed criteria for referral and evaluation of children for epilepsy surgery: recommendations of the subcommission for pediatric epilepsy surgery. Epilepsia 47: 952–9.
62. Daumas-Duport C, Scheithauer BW, Chodkiewicz JP, et al. (1988) Dysembryoplastic neuroepithelial tumor: A surgically curable tumor of young patients with intractable partial seizures: A report of thirty-nine cases. Neurosurgery 23: 545–56.
63. Daumas-Duport C, Varlet P, Bacha S, et al. (1999) Dysembryoplastic neuroepithelial tumors: non-specific histological forms: Study of 40 cases. J Neurooncol 41: 267–80.
64. Daumas-Duport C. (1993) Dysembryoplastic neuroepithelial tumors. Brain Pathol. 3: 283–95.
65. Honovar M, Janota I, Poekey CE. (1999) Histological heterogeneity of dysembryoplastic neuroepithelial tumor: Identification and differential diagnosis in a series of 74 cases. Histopathology 34: 342–56.
66. Lee DY, Chung CK, Hwang YS, et al. (2000) Dysembryoplastic neuroepithelial tumor: Radiological findings (including PET, SPECT, and MRS) and surgical strategy. J Neurooncol 47: 167–74.
67. Raymond AA, Halpin SFS, Alsanjari N, et al. (1994) Dysembryoplastic neuroepithelial tumor: Features in 16 patients. Brain 117: 461–75.
68. Raymond AA, Fish DR, Sisodiya SM, et al. (1995) Abnormalities of gyration, heterotopias, tuberous sclerosis, focal cortical dysplasia, microdysgenesis, dysembryoplastic neuroepithelial tumor and dysgenesis of the archicortex in epilepsy: Clinical, EEG, and neuroimaging features in 100 adult patients. Brain 118: 629–60.
69. Nolan MA, Sakuta R, Chuang N, et al (2004) Dysembryoplastic neuroepithelial tumors in childhood: Long-term outcome and prognostic features. Neurology 62: 2270–6.
70. Sandberg DI, Ragheb J, Dunoyer C, et al. (2005) Surgical outcomes and seizure control rates after resection of dysembryoplastic neuroepithelial tumors. Neurosurg Focus 18: E5.
71. Chan CH, Bittar RG, Davis GA, et al. (2006) Long-term seizure outcome following surgery for dysembryoplastic neuroepithelial tumor. J Neurosurg 104: 62–9.
72. Kameyana S, Fukuda M, Tomikawa M, et al. (2001) Surgical strategy and outcomes for epileptic patients with focal cortical dysplasia or dysembryoplastic neuroepithelial tumor. Epilepsia 42(Suppl 6): 37–41.
73. Sakuta R, Otsubo H, Nolan MA, et al. (2005) Recurrent intractable seizures in children with cortical dysplasia adjacent to dysembryoplastic neuroepithelial tumor. J Child Neurol 20: 377–84.
74. Valenti MP, Froelich S, Armspach JP, et al. (2002) Contribution of SISCOM imaging in the pre-surgical evaluation of temporal lobe epilepsy related to dysembryoplastic neuroepithelial tumors. Epilepsia 43: 270–6.
75. Degen R, Ebner A, Lahl R, et al. (2002) Various findings in surgically treated epilepsy patients with dysembryoplastic neuroepithelial tumors in comparison with those of patients with other low-grade brain tumors and other neuronal migration disorders. Epilepsia. 43: 1379–84.
76. Aronica E, Leenstra S, van Veelen CW, et al. (2001) Glioneuronal tumors and medically intractable epilepsy: A clinical study with long-term follow up of seizure outcome after surgery. Epilepsy Res 43:179–91.

77. Fomekong E, Baylac F, Moret C, et al. (1999) Dysembryoplastic neuroepithelial tumors. Analysis of 16 cases. Neurochirurgie 45: 180–9.
78. Hennessey MJ, Elwes RD, Binnie CD, et al. (2000) Failed surgery for epilepsy. A study of persistence and recurrence of seizures following temporal resection. Brain 123: 2445–66.
79. Kirkpatrick PJ, Honavar M, Janota I, et al. (1993) Control of temporal lobe epilepsy following en bloc resection of low-grade tumors. Neurosurgery 78: 19–25.
80. Prayson RA, Estes ML, Morris HH. (1993) Coexistence of neoplasia and cortical dysplasia in patients presenting with seizures. Epilepsia 34: 609–15.
81. Roach ES, Gomez MR, Northrup H. (1998) Tuberous sclerosis complex consensus conference: Revised clinical diagnostic criteria. J Child Neurol 13: 624–8.
82. Jambaque I, Chiron C, Dumas C, et al. (2000) Mental and behavioural outcome of infantile epilepsy treated by vigabatrin in tuberous sclerosis patients. Epilepsy Res 38: 151–60.
83. Cusmai R, Chiron C, Curotolo P, et al. (1990) Topographic comparative study of magnetic resonance imaging and electroencephalography in 34 children with tuberous sclerosis. Epilepsia 31: 747–55.
84. Ganji S, Hellman CD. (1985) Tuberous sclerosis: Long-term follow up and longitudinal electroencephalographic study. Clin Electroenceph 16: 219–24.
85. Pampiglione G, Moynahan EJ. (1976) The tuberous sclerosis syndrome: Clinical and EEG studies in 100 children. J Neurol Neurosurg Psychiatr 39: 666–73.
86. Westmoreland BF. (1988) Electroencephalographic experience at the Mayo clinic. In: Gomez HR (ed.). Tuberous sclerosis. New York: Raven Press, 37–49.
87. Jansen FE, Braun KPJ, van Nieuwenhuizen O, et al. (2003) Diffusion-weighted magnetic resonance imaging and identification of the epileptogenic tuber in patients with tuberous sclerosis. Arch Neurol 60: 1580–4.
88. Koh S, Jayakar P, Dunoyer C, et al. (2000) Epilepsy surgery in children with tuberous sclerosis complex: presurgical evaluation and outcome. Epilepsia 41: 1206–13.
89. Koh S, Jayakar P, Resnick TJ, et al. (1999) The localizing value of ictal SPECT in children with tuberous sclerosis and refractory partial epilepsy. Epileptic Disord 1: 41–6.
90. Rintahaka PJ, Chugani HT. (1997) Clinical role of positron emission tomography in children with tuberous sclerosis complex. J Child Neurol 12: 42–52.
91. Szelies B, Herholz K, Heiss WD, et al. (1983) Hypometabolic cortical lesions in tuberous sclerosis with epilepsy: demonstration by positron emission tomography. J Comput Assist Tomog 7: 946–53.
92. Asano E, Chugani DC, Chugani HT. (2003) Positron emission tomography. In: Curatolo P (ed.). Tuberous sclerosis complex: From basic science to clinical phenotypes. Cambridge: Cambridge University Press, 124–35.
93. Chugani DC, Chugani HT, Musik O, et al. (1998) Imaging epileptogenic tubers in children with tuberous sclerosis complex using $\alpha[^{11}C]$-methyl-L-tryptophan positron emission tomography. Ann Neurol 44: 858–66.
94. Juhasz C, Chugani DC, Musik O, et al. (2003) Alpha-methyl-L-tryptophan PET detects epileptogenic cortex in children with intractable epilepsy. Neurology 60:960–8.
95. Chandra PS, Salamon N, Huang J, et al. (2006) FDG-PET/ MRI coregistration and diffusion-tensor imaging distinguish epileptogenic tubers and cortex in patients with tuberous sclerosis complex: A preliminary report. Epilepsia 47: 1543–9.
96. Kamimura T, Tohyama J, Oishi M, et al. (2006) Magnetoencephalography in patients with tuberous sclerosis and localization-related epilepsy. Epilepsia 47: 991–7.
97. Jansen FE, Huiskamp G, van Huffelen AC, et al. (2006) Identification of the epileptogenic tuber in patients with tuberous sclerosis: A comparison of high-resolution EEG and MEG. Epilepsia 47: 108–14.
98. Romanelli P, Verdecchia M, Rodas R, et al. (2004) Epilepsy surgery for tuberous sclerosis. Pediatr Neurol 31: 239–47.
99. Bebin EM, Kelly PJ, Gomez MR. (1993) Surgical treatment for epilepsy in cerebral tuberous sclerosis. Epilepsia 34: 651–7.

100. Avellino AM, Berger MS, Rostomily RC, et al. (1997) Surgical management and seizure outcome in patients with tuberous sclerosis. J Neurosurg 87: 391–6.
101. Baumgartner JE, Wheless JW, Kulkarni S, et al. (1997) On the surgical treatment of refractory epilepsy in tuberous sclerosis complex. Pediatr Neurosurg 27: 311–8.
102. Guerreiro MM, Andermann F, Andermann A, et al. (1998) Surgical treatment of epilepsy in tuberous sclerosis: strategies and results in 18 patients. Neurology 51: 1263–9.
103. Thiele EA, Duffy FH, Poissaint TY. (2001) Intractable epilepsy and TSC: The role of epilepsy surgery in the pediatric population [Abstract]. J Child Neurol 16: 681.
106. Karenfort M, Kruse B, Freitag H, et al. (2002) Epilepsy surgery outcome in children with focal epilepsy due to tuberous sclerosis complex. Neuropediatrics 33: 255–61.
107. Vigliano P, Canavese C, Bobba B, et al. (2002) Transmantle dysplasia in tuberous sclerosis: Clinical features and surgical outcome in four children. J Child Neurol 17: 752–8.
108. Sinclair DB, Aronyk K, Snyder T, et al. (2003) Pediatric temporal lobectomy for epilepsy. Pediatr Neurosurg 38: 195–205.
109. Jarrar RG, Buchhalter JR, Raffel C. (2004) Long term outcome of epilepsy surgery in patients with tuberous sclerosis. Neurology 62: 479–81.
110. Lachhwani DK, Pestana E, Gupta A, et al. (2005) Identification of candidates for epilepsy surgery in patients with tuberous sclerosis. Neurology 64: 1651–4.
111. Weiner HL. (2004) Tuberous sclerosis and multiple tubers: Localizing the epileptogenic zone. Epilepsia 45(Suppl 4): 41–2.
112. Romanelli P, Weiner HL, Najjar S, et al. (2001) Bilateral resective epilepsy surgery in a child with tuberous sclerosis: case report. Neurosurgery 49: 732–5.
113. Quarato PP, Gennero GD, Manfredi M, et al. (2002) Atypical Lennox-Gastaut syndrome successfully treated with removal of a parietal dysembryoplastic tumor. Seizure 11: 325–9.
114. You SJ, Lee JK, Ko TS. (2007) Epilepsy surgery in a patient with Lennox-Gastaut syndrome and cortical dysplasia. Brain Dev 29: 167–70.
115. McKenzie RG. (1938) The present status of a patient who had the right cerebral hemisphere removed. JAMA 111: 168.
116. Krynauw RA. (1950) Infantile hemiplegia treated by removing one cerebral hemisphere. J Neurol Neurosurg Psychiatr 13: 243–67.
117. Rasmussen T. (1983) Hemispherectomy for seizures revisited. Can J Neurol Sci 10: 71–8.
118. Smith SJM, Andermann F, Villemure JG, et al. (1991) Functional hemispherectomy: EEG findings, spiking from isolated brain postoperatively, and prediction of outcome. Neurology 41: 1790–4.
119. Hoffman HJ, Hendrick EB, Dennis M, et al. (1979) Hemispherectomy for Sturge-Weber syndrome. Child Brain. 5: 233–48.
120. Graveline C, Mikulis D, Crawley AP, et al. (1998) Regionalized sensorimotor plasticity after hemispherectomy: fMRI evaluation. Pediatr Neurol 119: 337–42.
121. Graveline C, Hwang PA, Bone G, et al. (1999) Evaluation of gross and fine motor functions in children with hemidecortication: Prediction of outcome and timing of surgery. J Child Surg 14: 304–15.
122. Castroviejo IP, Diaz Gonzalez CD, Munoz-Hiraldo E. (1993) Sturge-Weber syndrome: A study of 40 patients. Pediatr Neurol 9: 283–7.
123. Cross JH. (2005) Neurocutaneous syndromes and epilepsy — issues in diagnosis and management. Epilepsia 46(Suppl 10): 17–23.
124. Hwang PA, Graveline C, Jay V, et al. (2001) The hemispheric epileptic disorders: Indications for hemispherectomy. In: Luders HO, Comair YG (eds.). Epilepsy surgery. Philadelphia: Lippincott Williams & Wilkins, 157–63.
125. Kossoff EH, Vining EPG, Pillas DJ, et al. (2003) Hemispherectomy for intractable unihemispheric epilepsy. Etiology vs outcome. Neurology 61: 887–90.
126. Jonas R, Nguyen S, Hu B, et al. (2004) Cerebral hemispherectomy. Hospital course, seizure, developmental, language, and motor outcome. Neurology 62: 1712–21.
127. Kossoff EH, Buck C, Freeman JM. (2002) Outcomes of 32 hemispherectomies for Sturge-Weber syndrome worldwide. Neurology 59: 1735–8.

128. Gonzalez-Martinez JA, Gupta A, Kotagal P, et al. (2005) Hemispherectomy for catastrophic epilepsy in infants. Epilepsia 46:1518–25.
129. Cook SW, Nguyen ST, Hu BS, et al. (2004) Cerebral hemispherectomy in pediatric patients with epilepsy: Comparison of three techniques by pathological substrate in 115 patients. J Neurosurg (Pediatrics 2) 100: 125–41.
130. Devlin AM, Cross JH, Harkness W, et al. (2003) Clinical outcomes of hemispherectomy for epilepsy in childhood and adolescence. Brain 126: 556–66.
131. Arzimanoglou AA, Andermann F, Aicardi J, et al. (2000) Sturge-Weber syndrome. Indications and results of surgery in 20 patients. Neurology 55: 1472–9.
132. Van Empelen R, Jennekens-Schinkel A, Buskens E, et al. (2004) Functional consequences of hemispherectomy. Brain 127: 2071–9.
133. Tinuper P, Andermann F, Villemure J-G, et al. (1988) Functional hemispherectomy for treatment of epilepsy associated with hemiplegia: Rationale, indications, results, and comparison with callosotomy. Ann Neurol 24: 27–34.
134. Delalande O, Fohlen M, Jalin C, et al. (2001) From hemispherectomy to hemispherotomy. In: Luders HO, Comair YG (eds.) Epilepsy surgery. Philadelphia: Lippincott Williams & Wilkins, 741–6.
135. O'Brien DF, Basu S, Williams DH, et al. (2006) Anatomical hemispherectomy for intractable seizures: Excellent seizure control, low morbidity and no superficial cerebral haemosiderosis. Child Nerv Syst 22: 489–98.
136. Villemure J-G. (2001) Functional hemispherectomy: Evolution of technique and results in 65 cases. In: Luders HO, Comair YG (eds.). Epilepsy surgery. Philadelphia: Lippincott Williams & Wilkins, 733–9.
137. Taylor DC, Neville BGR, Cross JH. (1997) New measure of outcome needed for the surgical treatment of epilepsy. Epilepsia 38: 625–30.

Section III
Psychosocial Issues

Chapter 10
Psychopathology in People with Epilepsy and Intellectual Disabilities

J. Dolman and M. Scheepers

Introduction

Psychopathology refers to the manifestation of behaviors or experiences that may be indicative of mental illness or psychological impairment. The term is broad, encompassing all phenomena that might, but might not, reach significance for a psychiatric diagnosis. As a result, the debate about the occurrence of psychopathology in people with epilepsy has been long and intense. If behavior is the manifest aspect of psychic life, then aberrations of behavior are usually attributed to some form of abnormal mental state[1]; there can be no doubt that this is a significant issue in people with epilepsy. There is further difficulty in interpreting psychopathology or behavioral disorders in people with intellectual disabilities (ID), particularly in people with severe ID. How, then, do we understand the issues surrounding psychopathology in people with ID and epilepsy?

In this chapter we will seek to look at these issues in more detail, describing findings in people with ID without epilepsy, in the general population with epilepsy, and then, where possible, looking for ID-specific research in the field of epilepsy.

Psychopathology in Intellectual Disability

Accurate measurement of psychopathology in any population can be difficult, but is made more difficult in people with ID because of methodological challenges. There is a need to define, appropriately, the terms to be used in research and this is especially important in this area.

In declaring an ID there is a need to, first and foremost, define the term. In most literature there is now agreement that ID is crudely defined by a significantly reduced ability to understand new or complex information, or to learn new skills, impaired intelligence (IQ below 70), and a reduced ability to manage independently (impaired social function), with onset in the developmental period (before the age of 18 years). Using this definition, between 2% and 3% of the general population

V.P. Prasher, M.P. Kerr (eds.) *Epilepsy and Intellectual Disabilities*,
DOI: 10.1007/978-1-84800-259-3_10, © Springer Science+Business Media, LLC 2008

will have ID, however, when epidemiological samples are collected, they seldom achieve more than a 0.5% ascertainment rate. The most likely reason for this is that most registers are based on the individual requiring a service (healthcare or social care) and therefore miss out on the majority who do not require, or are unaware of, services.[2] Most research in the field of ID therefore suffers from a sampling bias due to the nature of case ascertainment with an overrepresentation of people with more significant ID and a requirement for additional assistance. Because those people with mild ID are in contact with services, they are more likely to have a higher rate of psychopathology.

Defining psychopathology can be even more difficult than defining ID. Diagnostic and assessment tools should be applicable to people with ID. The World Health Organization's *International Classification of Diseases*, Tenth Edition (ICD-10)[3] and the American Psychiatric Association's *Diagnostic and Statistical Manual of Mental Disorders*, Fourth Edition (DSM-IV)[4] were designed for use in the general population. They rely on the subjective reporting of symptoms, and people with ID often do not recognize or cannot report their own symptoms. In addition, caregivers may not realize the significance of symptoms or overreport normal phenomena in people with ID. The Diagnostic Criteria for Adults with Learning Disability (DC-LD) attempts to address this issue.[5]

When the literature is reviewed, there is little consensus in terms of what may or may not be included. The terminology covered by the psychopathology rubric includes mental illness, mental disorder, psychiatric illness, psychiatric disorder, emotional problems, and behavioral problems. Some authors use the broad definitions in ICD-10,[3] DSM-IV,[4] or DC-LD,[5] while others wish to exclude behavior disorders and personality disorders when defining their research question. Often this will leave the reader pondering the research criteria and wondering whether the sample population presented represents the patients they see in clinical practice. Further difficulties arise when authors use a battery of assessment tools in order to define "caseness." These tools are not always comparable and seldom have relevance in a purely clinical setting, making it difficult for clinicians to apply the research to their practice. In addition, the method used for assessing psychopathology must be considered, as different prevalence rates can be found in the same

Table 10.1 Prevalence rates of mental illness

Disorder	Rate in ID(5)	Rate in General Population
Schizophrenia	3%	1%
Bipolar affective disorder	1.5%	1.2%
Depression	4%	3–7%
Generalized anxiety disorder	6%	3%
Specific phobia	6%	7%
Agoraphobia	1.5%	3.8%
Obsessive-compulsive disorder	2.5%	1.6%
Autism	7%	0.08%
Epilepsy	30%	1%

sample population, when diagnoses are compared using case notes, assessment tools, or clinical assessment.

About one in five people with ID have a behavior disorder, and this can account for as much as a third of referrals to specialist services. Within this group, there are some who will have a psychiatric diagnosis; however, a significant number will have a behavioral problem not immediately attributable to mental illness. It is therefore an important factor to consider when attributing causality.

The total prevalence of mental illness in people with ID is significantly greater than in the general population, particularly if behavioral and personality disorders are included. The lifetime prevalence probably lies between 30% and 50%

Psychopathology in Epilepsy in General Population

In research terms, there is a well-established relationship between epilepsy and behavior. However, research is often equivocal, with some repeat study findings not being replicated and in other studies, the opposite outcome found. The epidemiology of psychopathology in adults with epilepsy is poorly understood, partly because of ill-defined criteria, but also because of methodological problems. Most research is conducted from within specialist clinics, often university-based, where complex cases are managed with the most modern treatments and surgical options offered.[6] In these settings an increase in psychiatric morbidity has been established, but this should not be blandly accepted, as epilepsy is a chronic condition with a spectrum of severity and multiple etiological mechanisms.

Developmental Issues

Symptomatic epilepsies may result from a number of underlying pathological processes, which may be localized or diffuse, bilateral or unilateral, static or progressive; seizures may be the only apparent clinical manifestation. They may, however, also give rise to psychiatric deficits, the nature of which may depend on the nature, location, or time of injury to the developing brain.[1]

Children with epilepsy often do not attain parity, in education or employment, with their classmates. It has been suggested that attention deficits due to the epilepsy or to the antiepileptic drugs may be to blame; however, a study in a group of schoolchildren with idiopathic or cryptogenic epilepsy, who could expect normal educational and social development, ascertained that this was not the case. This case-controlled, longitudinal study found that children with newly diagnosed "epilepsy only" did not have persistent attention deficits and that antiepileptic drug (AED) treatment had no detrimental effect on attention, but prior school or behavioral difficulties and a maladaptive reaction from parents to the diagnosis of epilepsy, rather than epilepsy variables, were related to attentional deficits.[7] Further studies on the relationship between ID, epilepsy, and behavioral disorders have looked at the effect of medication on behavior, and no significant correlation between children taking antiepileptic medication and those not currently taking medication was found.[8]

Personality

Personality, and how it relates to chronic conditions, is a subject often evaluated, but results are seldom comparable or reproducible. This lack of consistency may be the result of a number of factors: the use of different tools in different studies, the validity of some of these tools in specific populations (people with epilepsy), the differences between patients with regards to social and psychological attitudes, and the problem with selection bias. Despite all of these possible reasons for skewed results, inconsistent findings have been reported when some control for these variables has occurred. This has led many clinicians to disregard personality traits in people with epilepsy; however, if we are to treat patients holistically, considering how these patients process information may be a key to improved quality of life and satisfaction with their interface with clinical services.[9]

Comorbidity of psychiatric and personality disorders has been associated with poorer response to treatment, lower compliance, and an increased risk of suicide. A recent study of patients with medically refractory epilepsy found 11 of 52 (21.15%) patients fulfilled research criteria for personality disorder. Dependent and avoidant personalities were the most common; the most frequent association with personality disorder was an epileptic aura. These results support previous reports of an increased rate of dependency and the social isolation associated with having epilepsy.[10]

Anxiety Disorders

Anxiety, phobias, and fear are common associations with the diagnosis of epilepsy, paroxysmal fear or anxiety being the most commonly reported aura (30%) in temporal lobe epilepsy (TLE). Because anxiety is a normal emotion and some anticipatory anxiety may be expected in people with a paroxysmal disorder that is not completely controlled, attention is not always given to anxiety disorders in the clinic setting. A disorder requires that impairment of social, occupational, and other areas of functioning occurs as a result of the anxiety.[9] Generalized anxiety disorders, panic disorder, phobias, and obsessive-compulsive disorder are conditions that exist in the general population, but may be amplified in people who also have epilepsy, particularly seizures arising from the temporal lobe.[11]

A comparison of patients with partial epilepsy (106 with TLE and 44 with frontal lobe epilepsy), idiopathic generalized epilepsy (70 patients), and controls demonstrated that there was a significant difference between anxiety and depression scores between the patients with epilepsy and the controls. In addition, patients with partial epilepsy scored higher than the idiopathic group, although this did not reach statistical significance. The previously reported association between left TLE and anxiety was replicated in this study but did not reach significance.[12]

Mood Disorders

Depression is the most common comorbid psychiatric condition associated with epilepsy, with a prevalence of up to 50% in patients with recurrent seizures and 10% in patients with controlled seizures.[13–17] It is generally underrecognized and undertreated and is incompletely understood, but it is thought to be the result of a combination of psychosocial and neurological factors. Although there is an association between chronic illness and depressive disorders, there seems to be an over-representation of depressive symptoms in patients with neurological disorders, and this is further increased if that neurological disorder includes epilepsy.[16]

Depression, it is argued, may not simply result from an understandable reaction to the difficulties of living with epilepsy; depression and epilepsy may in fact share common pathogenic mechanisms, including a shared genetic predisposition and neurotransmitter dysfunction with biogenic amines, gamma-amino-butyric acid (GABA), decreased metabolic and frontal lobe function all being implicated.[9,16,18] The seizures may themselves be involved, with suggested seizure-related variables including seizure type (complex partial seizures), location (temporal lobe), severity (increased depression rates with poorly controlled seizures), and laterality (left-sided focus) all being described.

Psychosocial factors, including perceived stigma, fear of seizures, discrimination, joblessness, and lack of social support have been implicated in the development of depressive disorders in people who have epilepsy. The relationship between psychosocial factors, depression, and epilepsy show that psychosocial variables are related to epilepsy, not just those people with epilepsy and depression.[19] When a psychosocial inventory was applied to a community sample of patients with epilepsy, it demonstrated that those no longer taking medication for their epilepsy were better adjusted than those who were on medication but who had had no seizures for a year, and this group was better adjusted than the group who were taking medication, but who had had a seizure in the past year. The authors conclude that the severity of epilepsy was associated with the severity of the self-reported psychosocial problems.[20]

Suicide, sudden unexpected death in epilepsy (SUDEP), accidents, and drowning are the most common cause of epilepsy-related death in people with epilepsy. With the advances in medication, status epilepticus is now less frequently registered as the cause of death in epilepsy in developed countries.[21] The suicide rate in epilepsy is fivefold higher than in the general population and is most significantly increased in patients with temporal lobe epilepsy (25-fold). Suicide appears to represent a serious problem to those attending specialist epilepsy clinics because they have more complex epilepsy.[21,22] In a retrospective analysis of suicide at a specialist epilepsy center, 10,739 patients were seen over a 12-year period. Five people completed suicide in this population. In an attempt to better understand why patients may have suicidal intent, the authors recognized an "interictal dysphoric disorder" (depressive mood, irritability, anxiety, headaches, insomnia, phobic fears, and anergia are prominent symptoms) which occurs independently of seizures, appears suddenly, and may last for hours to a couple of days. This mood disorder responds to antidepressant treatment, and the authors use a combination of treatments.[22] A second study of 1,722 patients attending an epilepsy center over a 14-year period revealed six completed suicides. The important findings were that suicide occurred soon after a seizure in patients with TLE, were more common in men, and were often related to psychotic episodes.[21]

Psychotic Phenomena

It has been noted for some time that psychosis is more common in people with epilepsy than in those without epilepsy and that within the epilepsy population it is more common in those with TLE. The prevalence of epilepsy and schizophrenia are both around 1%. It would be reasonable, therefore, to expect 1 in 100 patients with epilepsy to develop a schizophreniform psychosis; however, clinical studies have suggested a prevalence of around 3% in epilepsy, suggesting more than just a random association between the two disorders.[23]

Psychotic phenomena related to the seizure (ictal and postictal) are fairly clearly defined. **Ictal events** usually present with a delirium, are related to ongoing seizure activity, and respond to antiepileptic medication. **Postictal episodes** are discrete psychotic events occurring 24–48 hours after a cluster of seizures; they are short-lived (hours to days, sometimes up to a week); and occur in clear consciousness with hallucinations and delusions which are usually paranoid, often with a mystical or religious content. **Interictal psychoses** tend to have a more protracted (chronic) course, do not appear to be related to seizures, and often take the form of a schizophrenia-like illness.[24] Despite the similarities between chronic psychosis in epilepsy and schizophrenia, there are also significant differences. Patients with a chronic psychosis related to their epilepsy tend to demonstrate less formal thought disorder, less emotional withdrawal, fewer negative symptoms, no catatonia, and possibly a more favorable outcome after treatment.[25,26]

Risk Factors for Developing Psychosis

Numerous studies have looked at the risk factors for the development of psychosis in epilepsy. Unfortunately, results are not always consistent, and studies may be biased because of selection criteria. It is widely accepted that psychosis is more common in people with TLE (14%) compared with idiopathic generalized epilepsy (3.3%)[26]; however, recent studies have found no difference.[27,28] It is difficult to compare studies in the field because of the varying definitions of epilepsy, psychosis, and the risk factors identified, however, it is thought that female patients with TLE (complex partial seizures), with a left-sided focus on the electroencephalogram, will more commonly suffer from psychosis of epilepsy.[29] Recent studies have refuted this, with no difference being demonstrated in the sex, laterality of seizures, or age-related variables; rather, the associations found were related to level of intellectual functioning (more common in people with low or borderline ID) and family history (of psychosis but also mood disorder).[26,28]

Neuroimaging Studies

With the advances in neuroimaging and the ability to capture some "real-time" data, it is hoped that this field will illuminate some of the etiological processes that are held in the relationship between epilepsy and psychosis. A magnetic resonance imaging (MRI) study in patients with TLE and psychosis has identified potential structural differences in the brains of patients with temporal lobe epilepsy and psychosis as compared with TLE patients without psychopathology and healthy controls.[30] Twenty-six patients with psychosis in epilepsy (15 with postictal and 11 with interictal psychosis) were compared with 24 patients with epilepsy but without psychosis and 20 healthy controls. Findings in the group with psychosis showed smaller total brain volumes, significant bilateral amygdala volume enlargement (16–18%), but no difference in hippocampal volumes. When separately reviewed there was no difference between the groups with postictal or interictal psychosis.[24] A further MRI study compared a smaller sample (n=9) of patients with TLE with patients with schizophrenia and healthy controls.[31] The authors found that all patients had ventricular enlargement and a smaller temporal lobe, frontoparietal, and superior temporal gyrus volumes. These abnormalities were greatest in the group with psychosis of epilepsy. In five patients with TLE and postictal psychosis, single-photon emission computerized tomography scanning has demonstrated bifrontal and bitemporal hyperperfusion patterns during the psychosis. This reflects hyperactivation in these regions, and the authors suggest that this may be as a result of ongoing discharges, active inhibitory mechanisms involved in terminating seizures, or simply the dysregulation of cerebral blood flow.[32]

Psychiatric Symptomatology in TLE Patients

Studies in populations of individuals with schizophrenia have highlighted two symptom categories: positive and negative.[33] The latter negative group includes symptoms such as flattened affect and avolition and is associated with cognitive impairment. A study compared the presence of negative symptoms in 84 patients with TLE as compared with 74 healthy controls. Negative symptoms were significantly more prevalent (31%) in the TLE patients as compared to controls (8%). The population with negative symptoms had greater diffuse atrophy and higher cerebrospinal fluid volumes, as compared to both controls and TLE patients without negative symptoms. Negative symptoms were independent of past and current histories of depression.

Forced Normalization

Landolt described a group of patients who had productive psychotic episodes with forced normalization, the phenomenon characterized by the fact that, with the occurrence of the psychotic states, the EEG becomes more normal or entirely normal, as compared with previous or subsequent EEG findings. Tellenbach introduced the term "alternative psychosis," which described psychosis in epilepsy that had become controlled, but did not rely on EEG findings. This interesting phenomenon has, ever since, led to a burgeoning number of case reports but little in the line of formal research. Newer antiepileptic drugs and the emergence of behavioral changes with seizure freedom have led to a renewed interest in the field. Research is hampered by the conflicts and requirements: does the phenomenon require psychosis or will a behavioral change suffice, is near-normalization of the EEG a necessity or can the EEG findings be ignored? This has led to the development of diagnostic criteria, although these are not widely used or accepted.[34] It has been postulated that the phenomenon results from the suppression of cortical seizure-generating activity with seizure cessation and surface EEG normalization but secondary epileptogenesis and other linked phenomena (GABA, glutamate, and dopamine levels) that allow ongoing seizures to occur in the limbic areas with behavioral manifestations being predominant.[34]

Psychopathology and Epilepsy in ID Population

Despite epilepsy being the most common neurological disorder affecting people with ID, there are few studies, compared with the general population, that specifically present data on epilepsy, especially relating to psychopathology.[35] When reviewing and comparing the literature on psychopathology and epilepsy in people with ID it is important to take into consideration the following factors:

1. Identification and definition of ID
2. Identification of epilepsy and variables
3. Identification of populations and representativeness of study sample
4. Data analysis

Identification and Definition of ID

ID can be a state-dependent phenomenon (i.e., the person would not fulfill the criteria for ID were it not for some reversible variable) that may result from epilepsy or psychopathology. The first potential reversible variables relating to epilepsy include the ictal effects of subclinical seizures, focal discharges, postictal states, nonconvulsive status epilepticus, and the syndrome of electrical status epilepticus in sleep (ESES). The second relates to the drug-induced cognitive deficits particularly associated with phenobarbitone, phenytoin, sodium valproate, carbamazepine, and benzodiazepines.[36] The third variable relates to psychopathology, as individuals with serious mental health problems often score poorly on IQ assessments.[5] Although state-dependent ID would form only a small proportion of study participants, it acts as a reminder of how important it is to note whether studies have carefully examined the criteria for diagnosing an ID (applying the criteria of impaired intelligence, impaired social function, both occurring before the age of 18) if one is to apply research evidence to clinical practice.

Identification of Epilepsy and Variables

The International League Against Epilepsy (ILAE) has offered a classification system for epilepsy: in 1981 by seizure type and in 1989 by epilepsy syndrome. Good practice would suggest that epilepsy should be diagnosed at least at a level two (seizure type) but preferably at a level three (epilepsy syndrome) diagnosis.[37] It is important to differentiate between symptoms that arise in the interictal period (between seizures and not dependent on the seizure) and the periictal period (that arise as a result of the seizure).38 The instruments used in the measurement of symptoms should be specifically devised for the study of epilepsy within an ID population. Measures should not only take account of the seizure type/syndrome and seizure frequency, but also the patient's behavior, social interaction, independence, general well-being, and quality of life. In addition, they should be sensitive to change in psychopathology, and should pick up treatment compliance and environmental confounders, all of which present a significant challenge when studying people with ID.[36]

Identification of Populations and Representativeness of Study Samples

Most research data have effectively been collected from hospitals, institutions, psychiatric outpatients, and ID registers. Although this is helpful in informing us of the public health burden of any comorbidity, it is of little help in establishing causality and identifying risk in the wider community of people with ID. People recruited to these study populations are more likely to have psychiatric disorders, more severe epilepsy, more severe ID, and challenging behavior.[15,36] Adults with mild ID are more likely not to be known to ID services, and there is considerable variation in the methods used to set up and maintain ID registers, so they are not always comparable.

Data Analysis

As ID is, in itself, a risk factor for mental health problems, studies investigating psychopathology in people with ID and epilepsy are more likely to find increased prevalence rates when comparing with normative data from the general population (with and without epilepsy). Although it is helpful to understand the differences in presentation and prevalence between the psychopathology in people with ID compared with the general population, the relevance of psychopathology found in people with ID and epilepsy is only significant when compared with that found in people with ID who do not have epilepsy. It is therefore important that studies use assessment measures for which normative data are available or that they establish appropriately matched control groups.

In addition, the statistical methods should be appropriate and factors associated with only a relatively small proportion of variance should not be overemphasized.[39]

Rates of Psychopathology in People with ID and Epilepsy

Studies that used a control group generally found no statistically significant increase in the rate of psychopathology (psychiatric illness, behavioral problems, or personality disorder) between those with and without epilepsy.[38,39,43,55]

Psychiatric Disorders in People with ID and Epilepsy

A well-constructed study using the Psychiatric Assessment Schedule for Adults with Developmental Disabilities (PAS-ADD) Checklist found that 33% of the study population of people with ID and epilepsy met criteria for a possible psychiatric disorder. At the time of the study, no normative data were available for the PAS-ADD checklist; the authors therefore compared this data with data from two previous studies (one unpublished and one published) with similar demographics. In the former, 19% of participants had a possible psychiatric disorder and in the latter, 33%. However, any comparisons should be performed with caution, as all the data were potentially influenced by sampling factors.[55] In addition the PAS-ADD checklist used is primarily intended as a screening schedule to indicate whether further

Table 10.2 Summarizes the main studies investigating psychopathology in people with ID and epilepsy

Study	Reference Number	Authors	Population	Control	% mild ID	Psychopathology Studied	Assessment Tools	Results
1.	40	Lund (1985)	Institutions and community	None	Not stated	Psychiatric illness, which included autism and behavior disorder	Medical Research Council Schedule of Handicaps, Behaviours and Skills, Schedule of Psychiatric Symptoms	52% those with epilepsy (39% of this figure behavior disorder), 26% those without (SS).
2.	41	Espie CA, Pashley AS, Bonham KG, et al. (1989)	Hospital for people with ID	Matched pair comparison to those without epilepsy	<7%	Adaptive skills Behavioral disturbance	Adaptive Behaviour Scale, Psychosocial Behaviour Scale	People with epilepsy had poorer life skills. No difference with behavioral disturbance (SS).
3.	42	Gillies JB, Espie CA, Montgomery JM. (1989)	Attended day centers for people with ID.	Individually matched control group from same population without epilepsy	Most mild or moderate ID	Psychosocial functioning, including behavioral problems	Psychosocial Behaviour Scale	People with epilepsy had greater overall psychosocial dysfunction (SS).
4.	38	Deb S, Hunter D. (1991a)	Two hospitals and two day centers for people with ID	Individually matched control group from same population without epilepsy	1/3	Maladaptive behavior	The Profile of Abilities and Adjustment Schedule	Overall no difference between those with and without epilepsy (SS).

(continued)

Table 10.2 (continued)

Study	Reference Number	Authors	Population	Control	% mild ID	Psychopathology Studied	Assessment Tools	Results
5.	43	Deb S, Hunter D. (1991b)	Two hospitals and two day centers for people with ID	Individually matched control group from same population without epilepsy	1/3	Psychiatric illness	The Profile of Abilities and Adjustment Schedule, Present State Examination, clinical observation, DSM-III-R	47% those without epilepsy, 29%, those with (SS).
6.	44	Deb S, Hunter D. (1991c)	Two hospitals and two day centers for people with ID	Individually matched control group from same population without epilepsy	1/3	Personality disorder	The Standardised Assessment of Personality (SAP), The T-L Personal Behavior Inventory	No difference on SAP between those with and without epilepsy (SS). T-L score higher in those with epilepsy compared to those without if in community, receiving polypharmacy or have active epilepsy (SS).
7.	45	Deb S. (1994)	Two hospitals and two day centers for people with ID	Individually matched control group from same population without epilepsy	1/3	Maladaptive behavior, Psychiatric illness, Personality disorder	The Profile of Abilities and Adjustment Schedule, DSM-III-R, The Standardised Assessment of Personality.	No difference between those with and without epilepsy (SS).

8.	46	Deb S. (1995)	Institution and community settings	None	37%	Psychopathology and relationship to different EEG abnormalities	The Profile of Abilities and Adjustment Schedule, DSM-III-R, The Standardised Assessment of Personality.	No difference in psychopathology between pts whose EEG showed generalized and those with focal epileptiform changes (SS).
9.	47	Deb S. (1997)	Two hospitals and two day centres for people with ID	Individually matched control group from same population	1/3	Maladaptive behavior, Psychiatric illness, Personality disorder	The Profile of Abilities and Adjustment Schedule, ICD-9, The Standardised Assessment of Personality.	No difference for maladaptive behavior (SS). People without epilepsy more likely to suffer with psychiatric illness (SS). None for personality disorder (SS).
10.	48	Andrews TM, Everitt AD, Sander JWAS. (1999)	Long-term residents at National Epilepsy Centre	None	80% mild ID	Maladaptive behavior and relationship to MRI abnormalities	Aberrant Behaviour Checklist	Hyperactivity and non-compliance higher in those without focal lesions and with generalized epilepsy syndromes (SS).

(continued)

Table 10.2 (continued)

Study	Reference Number	Authors	Population	Control	% mild ID	Psychopathology Studied	Assessment Tools	Results
11.	49	Matson J, Bamburg JW, Mayville EA, et al., (1999)	Large residential facility in USA	None	Only 1% or less.	Social skills, adaptive skills, psychopathology, aberrant behaviors	Questions about Behavioural Function, Diagnostic Assessment for the Severely Handicapped, Aberrant Behaviour Checklist, The Matson Evaluation of Social Skills in Individuals with Severe Retardation, Vineland Adaptive Behaviour Scales Interview Form	People with epilepsy showed less social skills, adaptive skills, aberrant behavior and psychopathology than those without (SS).
12.	50	Chung MC, Cassidy G. (2001)	Hospital for people with ID	Matched pairs	Not stated, but for those with epilepsy <1/4 could wash and dress themselves and only 11% could understand	Challenging behavior	Disability Assessment Schedule, Aberrant Behaviour Checklist	Patients with epilepsy were more irritable than those without (SS).

13.	51	Espie CA, Watkins J, Curtice L, et al. (2003)	Hospital-based epilepsy clinics, specialist clinics for people with epilepsy and ID, and community learning disability teams. Only 14% lived in institutional setting.	Intragroup correlational design	25%	Psychiatric disorders, behavioral problems	Vineland Adaptive Behaviour Scales Interview Form, PAS-ADD Checklist	33% met criteria for possible psychiatric disorder, particularly affective/neurotic (see main text for discussion). Behavioral problem levels lower than population norms.
14.	52	Matsuura M, Oana Y, Kato A, et al. (2003)	All referrals to nine specialized epilepsy clinics in Japan	None	Not stated	Psychiatric disorders including personality disorders and mental retardation	Previous scheme devised by authors including ICD-10 guidelines	ID risk factor for psychopathology when compared to other patients with epilepsy (SS).
15.	53	Cowley A, Holt G, Bouras N, et al. (2004)	New referrals to specialist mental health service for people with ID	None	63%	Psychiatric diagnosis, excluding behavioral disorders	Assessment and information rating profile, ICD-10	Presence of epilepsy significantly associated with lower incidence of psychopathology.
16.	54	Matsuura M, Adachi N, Muramatsu K, et al. (2005)	All referrals to nine specialized epilepsy clinics in Japan	None	Not stated	Psychiatric, esp. psychotic disorders	Previous scheme devised by authors including ICD-10 guidelines	ID as risk factor for psychiatric and psychotic disorders compared to other patients with epilepsy (SS).

SS = statistically significant, Note: studies 4,5,6,7,9 conducted on same population sample.

mental health assessment may be required.[39] Normative data for the PAS-ADD Checklist have now been published, showing the prevalence rate to be 20.1%, suggesting there might be an increased rate of psychiatric symptoms in people with epilepsy.[5]

Four studies have suggested that the rate of psychiatric illness is lower in those with epilepsy compared to those people with ID only (numbers 4, 8, 10, and 14 from Table 10.2). When psychiatric illness was present, affective/neurotic disorder was the most prevalent category both in people with and without epilepsy (studies 4 and 12). However, people with epilepsy showed more schizophrenia and delusional disorder than those without epilepsy and, interestingly, no cases of bipolar affective disorder were found among those with epilepsy (study 4). In people with epilepsy, one study demonstrated a higher rate of changeable mood, but this did not reach statistical significance.[38]

When people with ID and epilepsy were compared with people with epilepsy but no ID, the two most frequent psychiatric disorders in those with ID and epilepsy were psychosis and personality disorders, while neurotic and psychotic disorders were most commonly found in those with epilepsy but no ID.

Personality Disorders

There are few studies specifically investigating the relationship between epilepsy and personality disorders in people with ID. Those that have been performed do not support the hypothesis that personality disorder is related to epilepsy in general, but further research is needed.[44]

Behavioral Problems

We know that behavioral problems are common in people with ID. There is still considerable debate over the effect that epilepsy and the antiepileptic drugs have on behavior in people with ID and epilepsy. Some studies have tried to establish whether there are relationships; many have simply described phenomena; few have actively looked at behavior before or after treatment; and most suffer the same selection bias that is pervasive in studies of people with ID.

In one study, people with active epilepsy were considered to be less cooperative and more echolalic than their matched, non-epilepsy-controlled peer group, and there were statistically significant differences between inpatients and people in the community who had epilepsy and ID. Inpatients were more likely to show less aggression if they only had single seizures rather than seizure clusters; less aggression and irritability when their EEG only showed background slow waves; more irritability if the EEG showed generalized epileptiform activity; and less aggression when on monotherapy, particularly carbamazepine. People in the community population with mild ID showed more destructive behavior and irritability; more aggression, and self-injury if the epilepsy was less than 20 years in duration; and, in addition, they showed more self-injury with multiple and frequent seizures.[43]

A further study, using the Aberrant Behaviour Checklist (ABC), demonstrated that the profiles of those with epilepsy and ID were similar to the standardization sample (used in the development of the ABC). Those with possible psychiatric disorder had higher scores for irritability, hyperactivity, and inappropriate speech, leading the authors to conclude that psychiatric status and behavior disorder are not necessarily independent of each other.[55]

In summary, the evidence that epilepsy, per se, increases the risk for the development of psychopathology in people with ID remains inconclusive. However, some epilepsy-specific factors may predict psychiatric disorder, and general factors, more closely associated with the disability, may be stronger predictors of behavioral problems.[55]

The Nature of the Combination of Psychopathology and Epilepsy in People with ID

Although much has been written about the relationship between psychopathology and epilepsy in the general population, there is still considerable variability at the individual level.[56] This variability is further increased when considering psychopathology in epilepsy in people with ID, since the nature of the combination of epilepsy, psychiatric disorder, and ID is complex and even less well understood. In addition, the population with ID is by no means homogeneous. The biopsychosocial model is often used to describe risk factors in the general population, and this is worth expanding in the population with ID to include the following[57]:

1. General effects resulting from the ID
2. Genetics/specific etiologies of the ID and epilepsy
3. The effects of seizures themselves
4. The psychosocial environment of the person
5. The effect of the treatment for the seizures

General Effects from the ID

People with epilepsy who also have ID have higher frequencies of slow wave EEG activity, a history of brain damage, and abnormal computerized tomography (CT) and MRI findings than people without ID.[54] In studies finding higher rates of psychiatric disorder in people with epilepsy and ID versus people with epilepsy but without ID, these dominant organic features are frequently cited as the cause. However, in a study where underlying brain damage was a predominant feature (i.e., severe ID and slow wave EEG activity) people with epilepsy had fewer problem behaviors than those without epilepsy but with ID.[43]

Persons with moderate ID and epilepsy were found to have significantly increased hyperactivity, noncompliance, and inappropriate speech scores than those with mild ID.[48] This, at face value, is supported by the findings that maladaptive behavior was associated with severe speech impediment, lower mood, excessive irritability, and less cooperativeness, although there was no significant difference in people with or without epilepsy.[35] General disability factors such as level of intellectual, sensory, or motor disability and side effects of medication contributed more to explaining behavioral problems than did epilepsy.[55]

While considering the general effect of the ID it may be important to consider the following hypothesis. Poorer attention and verbal factors are described in patients with epilepsy and psychosis compared with controls; this suggests that psychotic disorders in epilepsy are associated with underlying cognitive defects. Extrapolating this further, verbal dysfunction and attentional deficits may therefore result in a reduced capacity to deal with complex social problems, predisposing people with epilepsy to psychotic disorders.[54]

Genetics-Specific Etiologies of the ID and Epilepsy

Angelman Syndrome

Angelman syndrome is an uncommon genetic disorder, maternally inherited, and characterized by global developmental delay, unprovoked bursts of laughter, and frequent but brief epileptic seizures — atypical absences, tonic, atonic, and infrequent tonic-clonic. The individuals develop no meaningful expressive speech. Additional psychopathology seen includes autistic features, attention deficit syndrome, sleep disturbance, and stereotypical hand movements.[25,58]

Down Syndrome (DS)

Epilepsy occurs in 5–10% of people with DS and has a bimodal age distribution for seizure onset. The first peak is during childhood and presents as infantile spasms, myoclonic, atonic, and tonic-clonic seizures. Partial seizures are rarely seen,[25] and the second peak is in later life, usually as myoclonic or tonic-clonic seizures. Adults with DS and epilepsy do not have significantly greater maladaptive behaviors.[59] However, adaptive behavior skills can decline in adults with DS who develop epilepsy in later life, suggesting an association with dementia in Alzheimer's disease.[60]

Fragile X

Individuals have severe ID. In addition, boys with fragile X show delayed speech, echolalia, repetitive speech, hand flapping, and attentional deficits.[61] Epilepsy (infantile spasms, tonic-clonic, and atonic seizures) occurs in 30–40% of patients, usually presenting in childhood.[25] Twenty-five percent of persons with fragile X have autism, and many more people with fragile X have a behavioral phenotype that does not fulfill the full criteria for autism.

Landau-Kleffner Syndrome

This is a rare disorder based on clear clinical and EEG criteria, with onset between the ages of three and eight years. Half of patients present with verbal agnosia (severe impairment or loss of verbal and auditory understanding) and expressive aphasia, and half with seizures. Of the former group, 20–30% develop seizures weeks or months after the initial speech symptoms. During wakefulness the EEG shows typical multifocal slow, spike, and spike-wave discharge in the temporal or centrotemporal regions. During sleep there are bursts of prolonged slow, spike-slow wave discharges, which may be focal but are commonly generalized and can last for several hours. Behavioral disturbances are common, and although they may be due to the frustration resulting from the speech impairment, the very frequent abnormal interictal EEG activity, particularly during sleep, or the as yet unknown underlying etiology may contribute.[25]

Lennox-Gastaut Syndrome

This is a common epilepsy syndrome, characterized by multiple seizure types (tonic, prolonged atypical absence, atonic, and tonic-clonic seizures), characteristic EEG findings (frequent paroxysms of slow, spike and slow wave activity, fast spiking activity, and nonconvulsive status), and almost invariably severe ID. An earlier age of onset may be associated with a specific cause, e.g., West syndrome, whereas later-onset cases are more likely to be classified as cryptogenic. Children can show evidence of frontal lobe dysfunction – limited attention span, poor judgment, no sense of danger, impulsivity, and grossly disinhibited verbal and physical behavior. This may be due to the frequent seizures (including unrecognized nonconvulsive status epilepticus), frequent or continuous EEG activity in sleep, the underlying cause of the syndrome, and cumulative effects of head injuries from tonic and atonic seizures and AEDs.[25]

Lesch-Nyhan Syndrome

Lesch-Nyhan syndrome is an X-linked syndrome, almost exclusive to males in which 50% of individuals suffer with seizures, moderate ID, and compulsive self-injury.

Rett Syndrome

This is an uncommon genetic disorder specifically affecting girls (the disorder is thought to be fatal in male fetuses), which, prior to the discovery of the genetic basis for the disorder, was probably misdiagnosed as autism. A period of normal development (18 months) is followed by a severe decline in functional ability and the development of stereotypic behaviors and epilepsy. There are different diagnostic EEG patterns at different stages during the period of loss of ability. Epilepsy develops in early childhood, usually in the form of complex partial, atypical absence, and tonic-clonic seizures, but often these seizures diminish by adolescence. Adults are severely disabled with frequent symptoms of depression, anxiety, self-injury, and panic.[25,58]

Tuberous Sclerosis (TS)

Seizures occur in 65% of people with TS, often presenting as infantile spasms. The likelihood of an ID is greatest in children who have infantile spasms and uncontrolled seizures.[62] In addition to a general delay in development, individuals can have language, reading, and spelling disorders. Autism is reported in 25%, and a more broad diagnosis of pervasive developmental disorder in 50%. Fifty percent to 60% of individuals show disruptive behavior characterized by marked hyperactivity and attention deficits. Children may also have problems with sleep, aggression, and self-injury.[63]

Velo-Cardio-Facial Syndrome

This is one of the most common genetic disorders caused by deletion of a small segment of the long arm of chromosome 22. Among the features found in people who have this syndrome are seizures, mild ID, attention deficit disorder, mood disorders, psychotic disorders, social immaturity, obsessive compulsive disorder, generalized anxiety disorder, phobias, and a severe startle response. Since the list of psychiatric/psychological symptoms includes almost all diagnoses it is difficult to know without further research whether the findings are incidental as a result of this being one of the most common genetic disorders.[64]

Miscellaneous Etiologies

Disorders of neuronal migration (lissencephaly, polymicrogyria, pachygyria) and metabolic disorders present across the range of epilepsies and levels of ID, and may be due to a variety of etiologies. Many of the more malignant epilepsy syndromes that are associated with ID are termed "epileptic encephalopathies," as any cognitive impairment or ID is considered to be directly related not only to the frequency of the clinical seizures but also through the very frequent, if not at times persistent, abnormal interictal (subclinical) paroxysmal (epileptiform) activity recorded on the EEG.[25]

No specific research has explored psychopathology in these epilepsy syndromes; however, any studies that include people with ID and epilepsy will inevitably include such individuals.

The Effects of Seizures Themselves

"Disturbed behavior is not associated with epilepsy per se... a small sub-group of subjects who have poorly controlled epilepsy do present greater behavioral problems."[41]

Once again the research evidence in this area is contradictory. The association between psychopathology and location of seizure activity in the brain does not appear to be significant in people with ID; however, inappropriate speech has been associated with simple partial seizures,[50] a higher frequency of hyperactivity and noncompliance behavior was found in people with generalized epilepsy syndromes but no focal lesion on MRI,[48] and an increased rate of problem behaviors in those with generalized activity on the EEG has been described.[38] In fact, a past history of febrile convulsions (which is strongly associated with mesial temporal sclerosis on MRI in later life), although found to be associated with increased irritability and agitation, was not associated with MRI changes.[48]

Increased seizure activity (i.e., multiple seizure types, high frequency and severity) appears to be an important predictor of psychosocial dysfunction and behavior disturbance.[41,42,43,50,51] The evidence for psychiatric illness is contradictory, with greater psychiatric disorder being significantly associated with both greater seizure severity and a greater number of seizures in the past month[55] and less psychiatric illness with more active epilepsy, an earlier age of onset, longer duration of epilepsy and more frequent seizures both being described.[38] A reduced tendency to loss of consciousness during seizures (partial seizures) is a particular risk factor for psychiatric disorder. Although loss of consciousness is a symptom of generalized epilepsy, a more plausible explanation may be that seizures involving loss of consciousness may be experienced as less distressing.[55]

The Psychosocial Environment of the Person

The many confounding variables that make research on the influence of psychosocial/environmental factors on psychopathology in people with epilepsy difficult are summed up by the paucity of studies completed in this field. The finding that significantly more destructive behavior and irritability occurred in mild and moderate ID patients with epilepsy residing in the community, compared with those in hospital, suggests that psychosocial factors do play a role in the development of psychopathology, as this influence would be less prominent in people with severe ID or hospitalized patients.[43]

If the research conducted in the general population is to be extrapolated into ID, one can assume that these factors play a significant role, as the important factors include early onset of seizures, increased life events in the past year, financial stress and employment difficulties, social exclusion and stigma, an external locus of control, and poor adjustment to epilepsy.[65] There is certainly evidence that the first four factors in this list are significant in people with ID.

The Effect of the Treatment

There are now a number of AEDs licensed for the management of epilepsy. Each drug has a specific indication, some have a broad spectrum of action (partial and generalized seizures), and some may be more specific (partial seizures only). There is a wealth of guidance on the appropriate management of epilepsy; most guidance recommends a single drug (monotherapy) where possible, however, some refractory epilepsy may require the use of more than one drug (polytherapy). In those people with uncontrolled seizures and polytherapy there is a consistent and significant increased risk of behavioral disturbance, independent of seizure frequency.[41,51] A couple of reasons make polytherapy likely to interfere with social and educational opportunities. First, any behavioral disorders associated with polytherapy may cause placement difficulties, limiting the opportunity for the individual to develop social awareness, competence, and feelings of control. Second, the combined side effect profiles often raise the likelihood of drug toxicity and sedation. The limited social and educational opportunities may cause a failure to acquire adaptive interpersonal and life skills, which may result in further behavior problems and a cycle of repeated social failure in which epilepsy and AEDs are major components.[42,51] A significant decrease in the intrusiveness of problematic behaviors may result from a reduction of polytherapy.[66]

Methodological problems and the risk of confounding factors result in AED side effects and their relationship with psychopathology in people with ID not being well described. Among the problems, caregiver reporting and the high level of pretreatment behaviors are often cited as uncontrollable variables. However, side effects could be an explanatory factor for inappropriate speech and irritability,[55] and the sedative effect of AEDs may explain why psychiatric illness was less frequent in people with more active epilepsy, but this does not explain the increase in behavioral problems in people with more active epilepsy in the same study.[38]

Barbiturates, especially phenobarbitone, may provoke hyperkinetic syndromes,[40] and its sedating effect is known to adversely alter psychosocial functioning.[51] The difficulties associated with the side effect profiles of phenobarbitone and phenytoin result in their use in people with ID and epilepsy not being recommended.[67] Carbamazepine is thought to have less cognitive and behavioral side effects than other AEDs as a result of the mood stabilizing effect.[43,51] However, more recent studies comparing it with modern drugs show that it is cognitively impairing and can cause significant problems on initiation.[68] Modern AEDs are usually well tolerated and free of significant problems if used appropriately. There are a number of reports of behavioral effects relating to the newer drugs, but these need to be interpreted with care. Benzodiazepines are sedating and may be associated with paroxysmal released aggression. Tiagabine has been reported to have dose-related anxiety effects, and topiramate may cause significant side effects if escalated quickly.[68] Lamotrigine, although having a positive cognitive side effect profile, can be too stimulating for some people with ID, which causes problems for the caregivers. Vigabatrin may cause visual field defects in up to 50% of users and has an association with psychosis in the general population and behavioral disturbance in people with ID.[68]

All AEDs may cause the phenomenon of "forced normalization" with a concomitant deterioration of mental state when seizures are well controlled. This has not been extensively studied in people with ID, although in clinical practice, the phenomenon is often used to describe behavior changes in children with ID and epilepsy when their seizures improve. Serum folate levels are known to be reduced by some AEDs, and it has been postulated that there may be an association with reduced folate levels and psychiatric illness, personality disorder, and behavioral problems in people with ID; however, this has been discounted.[46]

Conclusion

Psychopathology is a broadly defined term that researchers use to describe a host of phenomena that include behavioral, personality, and psychiatric disorders. People with ID do not form a homogeneous or particularly well-studied group. Significant methodological problems remain in this research field, and it is not always easy to translate research findings into clinical practice.

There is clear evidence that psychopathology, in its broadest sense (including behavioral, personality, and psychiatric disorders), is a common feature in people with ID. Due to the methodological flaws, the ID study populations described are likely to be representative of the people seen in clinical practice, as they make up the people known to services. The difficulty is in generalizing the information from these studies or comparing the evidence with the general population. The inherent difficulties in diagnosing psychopathology (communication, self-reporting, caregiver expectation, stigma) in people with ID should not get in the way of using appropriate tools and classification systems in order to appropriately treat psychopathology when it occurs. In the general population with epilepsy, there seems to be a higher rate of psychopathology than would be expected. If we consider a biopsychosocial approach to the question, we can see there are variables in each of the domains. Anxiety, mood disorders (particularly dysthymia), and psychosis are all described as being related to the seizures themselves or may occur in the period immediately following the seizures. There are some elegant theories and interesting hypotheses on the reasons for this, and there is hope that more up to date imaging and some real-time visual feedback will result in a better understanding of the relationship between seizures and psychiatric phenomena. The psychological and social aspects of epilepsy and their contribution to the development of psychopathology are less well studied but nonetheless are responsible for a considerable addition to the burden of suffering with epilepsy.

The overall conclusion remains that both behavioral and psychiatric disorders, whatever reasonable definitions are used, are common in people with intellectual disability and epilepsy. The relationship between psychopathology and epilepsy is less well understood, but it seems that it is largely factors other than the epilepsy itself that are responsible for the high prevalence. There are specific factors relating to the intellectual disability per se, these include specific behavioral phenotypes, which may occur in the presence of epilepsy but are not dependent on it being present. Where epilepsy is present, it is important to consider all possibilities rather than to simply discount the symptoms as part of the overall condition.

When managing epilepsy in people with ID it is important to note any baseline psychopathology at the first visit. If, during the course of treatment, psychopathology is found, it is important to try to classify it using an appropriate system. If this achieves a level of significance that requires further intervention, it is important to consider which elements may be contributing to the disorder: the individual, the etiology of the ID, the environment, the epilepsy, and/or the medication. None of these should preclude the individual from appropriate treatment if this is required.

References

1. Engel J, Taylor DC. (1997) Neurobiology of behavioural disorders. In: Engel J, Pedley TA (eds.). Epilepsy — A comprehensive textbook. Philadelphia: Lippincot-Raven, 2045–52.
2. Tymchuk AJ, Lakin KC, Luckasson R. (2001) Life at the margins: Intellectual, demographic, economic, and social circumstances of adults with mild cognitive limitations. In: Tymchuk AJ, Lakin KC, Luckasson R (eds.). The forgotten generation: The status and challenges of adults with mild cognitive limitations. Baltimore: Paul H.Brookes.
3. World Health Organization. (1992) The ICD-10 Classification of mental and behavioural disorders. Clinical descriptions and diagnostic guidelines. Geneva: WHO.
4. American Psychiatric Association. (1995) Diagnostic and statistical manual of mental disorders, Third Edition Revised. (DSM-IV) Washington, DC.
5. Smiley E. (2005) Epidemiology of mental health problems in adults with learning disability: An update. Adv Psychiatr Treatment 11: 214–22.
6. Hermann B, Whitman S. (1992) Psychopathology in epilepsy. The role of psychology in altering paradigms of research, treatment, and prevention. Am Psychol 47: 1134–8.
7. Oostrom KJ, Schouten A, Kruitwagen CL, et al. (2002) Attention deficits are not characteristic of schoolchildren with newly diagnosed idiopathic or cryptogenic epilepsy. Epilepsia 43: 301–10.
8. Lewis JN, Tonge BJ, Mowat DR, et al. (2000) Epilepsy and associated psychopathology in young people with intellectual disability. J Paediatr Child Health 36: 172–5.
9. Scheepers M, Kerr M. (2003) Epilepsy and behaviour. Curr Opin Neurol. 16: 183–7.
10. Lopez-Rodriguez F, Altshuler L, Kay J, et al. (1999) Personality disorders among medically refractory epileptic patients. J Neuropsychiatr Clin Neurosci 11: 464–9.
11. Marsh L, Rao V. (2002) Psychiatric complications in patients with epilepsy: A review. Epilepsy Res 49: 11–33.
12. Piazzini A, Canger R. (2001) Depression and anxiety in patients with epilepsy. Epilepsia 42(Suppl 1): 29–31.
13. Bortz JJ. (2003) Neuropsychiatric and memory issues in epilepsy. Mayo Clin Proc. 78: 781–7.
14. Gilliam F, Kanner AM. (2002) Treatment of depressive disorders in epilepsy patients. Epilepsy Behav 3(5S)2–9.
15. Brookes G, Crawford P. (2002) The associations between epilepsy and depressive illness in secondary care. Seizure 11: 523–6.
16. Barry JJ. (2003) The recognition and management of mood disorders as a comorbidity of epilepsy. Epilepsia 44(Suppl 4): 30–40.
17. Kanner AM. (2003) Depression in epilepsy: Prevalence, clinical semiology, pathogenic mechanisms, and treatment. Biol Psychiat. 54: 388–98.
18. Kanner AM, Balabanov A. (2002) Depression and epilepsy: How closely related are they? Neurology 58(8 Suppl 5): S27–S39.

19. Schmitz EB, Robertson MM, Trimble MR. (1999) Depression and schizophrenia in epilepsy: Social and biological risk factors. Epilepsy Res 35: 59–68.

20. Trostle JA, Hauser WA, Sharbrough FW. (1989) Psychologic and social adjustment to epilepsy in Rochester, Minnesota. Neurology. 39: 633–7.

21. Fukuchi T, Kanemoto K, Kato M, et al. (2002) Death in epilepsy with special attention to suicide cases. Epilepsy Res 51: 233–6.

22. Blumer D, Montouris G, Davies K, et al. (2002) Suicide in epilepsy: Psychopathology, pathogenesis, and prevention. Epilepsy Behav 3: 232–41.

23. McLachlan RS. (2003) Psychosis and epilepsy: A neurologist's perspective. Seishin Shinkeigaku Zasshi 105: 433–9.

24. Trimble MR, van Elst LT. (2003)The amygdala and psychopathology studies in epilepsy. Ann NY Acad Sci. 985: 461–8.

25. Appleton R. (2003) Aetiology of epilepsy and learning disorders: Specific epilepsy syndromes; genetic, chromosomal and sporadic syndromes. In: Trimble MR (ed.). Learning disability and epilepsy: An integrative approach. Guildford: Clarius Press, 47–64.

26. Alper KR, Barry JJ, Balabanov AJ. (2002) Treatment of psychosis, aggression, and irritability in patients with epilepsy. Epilepsy Behav 3(5S):13–18.

27. Onuma T. (2000) Classification of psychiatric symptoms in patients with epilepsy. Epilepsia 41(Suppl 9): 43–8.

28. Adachi N, Onuma T, Nishiwaki S, et al. (2000) Inter-ictal and post-ictal psychoses in frontal lobe epilepsy: A retrospective comparison with psychoses in temporal lobe epilepsy. Seizure 9: 328–35.

29. Trimble MR, Schmitz EB. (1997) The psychoses of epilepsy/schizophrenia. In: Engel J, Pedley TA (eds.). Epilepsy: A comprehensive textbook. Philadelphia: Lipincott-Raven, 2071–82.

30. Tebartz VE, Baeumer D, Lemieux L, et al. (2002) Amygdala pathology in psychosis of epilepsy: A magnetic resonance imaging study in patients with temporal lobe epilepsy. Brain 125: 140–9.

31. Marsh L, Sullivan EV, Morrell M, et al. (2001) Structural brain abnormalities in patients with schizophrenia, epilepsy, and epilepsy with chronic interictal psychosis. Psychiatr Res. 108: 1–15.

32. Leutmezer F, Podreka I, Asenbaum S, et al. (2003) Postictal psychosis in temporal lobe epilepsy. Epilepsia 44: 582–90.

33. Getz K, Hermann B, Seidenberg M, et al. (2002) Negative symptoms in temporal lobe epilepsy. Am J Psychiat 159: 644–51.

34. Krishnamoorthy ES, Trimble MR. (1999) Forced normalization: Clinical and therapeutic relevance. Epilepsia 40(Suppl 10): S57–S64.

35. Deb S. (1997) Mental disorder in adults with mental retardation and epilepsy. Compr Psychiat 38: 179–84.

36. Krishnamoorthy ES. (2003) Neuropsychiatric epidemiology at the interface between learning disability and epilepsy. In: Trimble MR (ed.). Learning disability in epilepsy: An integrative approach. Guildford: Clarius Press, 17–26.

37. Frost S, Crawford P, Mera S. (2002) National statement of good practice for the treatment and care of people who have epilepsy. Joint Epilepsy Council.

38. Deb S, Hunter D. (1991) Psychopathology of people with mental handicap and epilepsy. II. Psychiatric illness. Br J Psychiat 159: 826–4.

39. Besag FM. (2003) Psychopathology in people with epilepsy and intellectual disability. J Neurol Neurosurg Psychiat 74: 1464.

40. Lund J. (1985). Epilepsy and psychiatric disorder in the mentally retarded adult. Acta Psychiat Scand. 72: 557–62.

41. Espie CA, Pashley AS, Bonham KG, et al. (1989). The mentally handicapped person with epilepsy: A comparative study investigating psychosocial functioning. J Ment Defic Res 33: 123–35.

42. Gillies JB, Espie C, Montgomery J. (1989). The social and behavioural functioning of people with mental handicaps attending Adult Training Centres: A comparison of those with and without epilepsy. Ment Handicap Res 2: 129–36.

43. Deb S, Hunter D. (1991) Psychopathology of people with mental handicap and epilepsy. I. Maladaptive behaviour. Br J Psychiat 159: 822–4.

44. Deb S, Hunter D. (1991) Psychopathology of people with mental handicap and epilepsy. III. Personality disorder. Br J Psychiat 159: 830–4.

45. Deb S. (1994) Effect of folate metabolism on the psychopathology of adults with mental retardation and epilepsy. Am J Ment Retard. 98: 717–23.

46. Deb S. (1995) Electrophysiological correlates of psychopathology in individuals with mental retardation and epilepsy. J Intellect Disabil Res 39: 129–35.

47. Deb S. (1997) Mental disorder in adults with mental retardation and epilepsy. Compr Psychiat 37: 179–84.

48. Andrews TM, Everitt AD, Sander JW. (1999) A descriptive survey of long-term residents with epilepsy and intellectual disability at the Chalfont Centre: Is there a relationship between maladaptive behaviour and magnetic resonance imaging findings? J Intellect Disabil Res 43: 475–83.

49. Matson J, Bamburg JW, Mayville EA, et al. (1999) Seizure disorders in people with intellectual disability: An analysis of differences in social functioning, adaptive functioning and maladaptive behaviours. J Intell Dis Res 43: 531–9.

50. Chung MC, Cassidy G. (2001) A preliminary report on the relationship between challenging behaviour and epilepsy in learning disability. Eur J Psychiat 15: 23–32.

51. Espie CA, Gillies JB, Montgomery JM. (1990) Antiepileptic polypharmacy, psychosocial behaviour and locus of control orientation among mentally handicapped adults living in the community. J Ment Defic Res 34: 351–60.

52 Matsuura M, Oana Y, Kato M, et al. (2003). A multicenter study on the prevalence of psychiatric disorders among new referrals for epilepsy in Japan. Epilepsia. 44: 107–14.

53. Cowley A, Holt G, Bouras N, et al. (2004) Descriptive psychopathology in people with mental retardation. J Nerv Ment Dis 192: 232–7.

54. Matsuura M, Adachi N, Muramatsu R, et al. (2005) Intellectual disability and psychotic disorders of adult epilepsy. Epilepsia 46(Suppl 1):11–14.

55. Espie CA, Watkins J, Curtice L, et al. (2003) Psychopathology in people with epilepsy and intellectual disability: An investigation of potential explanatory variables. J Neurol Neurosurg Psychiat 74: 1485–92.

56. Hermann BP, Whitman S. (1991) Neurobiological, psychosocial, and pharmacological factors underlying interictal psychopathology in epilepsy. Adv Neurol 55: 439–52.

57. Pond DA. (1967) Behaviour disorders in brain-damaged children. Mod Trends Neurol 4: 125–34.

58. Berney T. (1997) Behavioural Phenotypes. In: Russell O (ed.). Seminars in the Psychiatry of Learning Disability. London: Gaskell, 63–80.

59. Prasher VP. (1995) Epilepsy and associated effects on adaptive behaviour in adults with Down syndrome. Seizure. 4:53–6.

60. Collacott RA. (1993) Epilepsy, dementia and adaptive behaviour in Down's syndrome. J Intellect Disabil Res 37: 153–60.

61. Turk J, Hill P. (1995) Behavioural phenotypes in dysmorphic syndromes. Clin Dysmorphol 4: 105–15.

62. O'Callaghan FJ, Harris T, Joinson C, et al. (2004) The relation of infantile spasms, tubers, and intelligence in tuberous sclerosis complex. Arch Dis Child. 89: 530–3.

63. Tuberous Sclerosis Association. (2002) Clinical guidelines for the care of patients with tuberous sclerosis complex: Summary.

64. The Velo-cardio-facial syndrome Education Foundation. (2006) Specialist fact sheet. http://www.vcfsef.org.

65. Hermann BP, Whitman S, Wyler AR, et al. (1990) Psychosocial predictors of psychopathology in epilepsy. Br J Psychiat 156: 98–105.

66. Fischenbacher E. (1982) Effect of reduction of anticonvulsants on wellbeing. Br Med J. 285: 423–4.

67. Clinical guidelines for the management of epilepsy in adults with an intellectual disability. (2001) Seizure 10: 401–9.

68. Kerr M. (2003) Anti-epileptic drug treatments in patients with learning disability. In: Trimble MR (ed.). Learning disability and epilepsy: An integrative approach. Guildford: Clarius Press, 141–60.

Chapter 11
Associated Physical Problems of Epilepsy in Intellectual Disabilities

C.L. Morgan

Introduction

It is well documented that people with intellectual disabilities (ID) have an excess prevalence of epilepsy. Various studies have reported a wide range of prevalence of epilepsy from between 14% and 44% for patients with an ID[1] compared to less than 1% in the population as a whole.[2] The risk of epilepsy in people with an ID is associated with both the severity of ID[3] and the specific underlying etiologies of ID, such as Down's syndrome (DS)[4] and cerebral palsy.[5] Consequently, there is the likelihood that patients with ID and with epilepsy will have increased physical health issues associated with this increased severity and type of ID, in addition to those physical morbidities and events associated with epilepsy, such as fractures and trauma and the side effects of antiepileptic medication.

Within the general population, the prevalence of epilepsy is highest among the older age groups. This is due to the onset of seizures as a sequelae to cerebrovascular events and other morbidities, such as cerebral tumors and Alzheimer's disease (AD). However, within the ID population the reverse of this relationship is true.[6] This results from the high incidence of epilepsy occurring from birth and within the early years of life and also from the higher mortality rates associated with both severity of ID[7,8] and specific underlying diagnoses such as DS.[9] Consequently, conditions associated with the aging process, such as cardiovascular disease and certain types of cancer, will be underrepresented in a crude comparison between those patients with ID and without epilepsy. In addition, conditions common among patients with epilepsy which underline their condition, such as cerebrovascular disease, will be far less common in the subset of people with epilepsy and coexisting ID.

The aim of this chapter is to highlight those conditions which are particularly relevant to patients with both ID and epilepsy. In particular it focuses upon those events and morbidities associated with epilepsy, such as injuries resulting from falls, burns, and drowning. As with many other areas of research into epilepsy within the context of the ID population, the specific literature is relatively scarce, with the result that extrapolations must be made from the general population with epilepsy.

V.P. Prasher, M.P. Kerr (eds.) *Epilepsy and Intellectual Disabilities*,
DOI: 10.1007/978-1-84800-259-3_11, © Springer Science + Business Media, LLC 2008

Injuries: Overview

The risk of injury for patients with epilepsy has been well documented.[10] Predominantly this risk is due to injuries occurring as a consequence of seizures. One United Kingdom (UK) study surveyed community patients and revealed that for those patients who had suffered a seizure in the previous year nearly one quarter had sustained a head injury, 16% had been burned, 10% had received dental injuries, and 6% had suffered a fracture.[11,12] Clearly this excess of injuries is largely explained by the impact of seizures themselves; there appears to be no increase between patients with and without epilepsy once seizure-related injuries are discounted.[13]

Patients with ID are also at twice the risk of injuries than the population in general, although this is specific to the nature of the injury and the setting. Whereas, for example, the risk of aspiration is greatly increased for people with ID and there are clear increases for falls and near drownings, injuries resulting from self-harm, assault, and transport are considerably less frequent. Injuries for people with ID are also more likely to occur at the person's usual residence (either home or in an institutional setting) rather than outside.[14]

For those patients with an ID and coexisting epilepsy, this well-described risk of injury remains. The risk of injury among patients with ID is doubled for those with coexisting epilepsy, and this is independent of other confounding factors, such as severity of disability and associated psychopathology.[14] A Norwegian study based on the prospective observation of 62 institutionalized patients over a 13-month period recorded a total of 6,889 seizures, of which just under 40% resulted in a fall. A total of 80 injuries was recorded, representing an injury rate per seizure of 1.2%, although the majority of these injuries were regarded as minor. A total of 59 injuries involved soft tissue injuries, mainly to the face. One patient, however, suffered a subdural hematoma and consequently died during an restorative operative procedure.[15] In the sections below, the risk of the specific injuries of burns, drowning, fractures, and trauma are considered for patients with ID and coexisting epilepsy.

Burns

Burn injuries occur more frequently in patients with epilepsy than in the general population. A study of 134 patients with epilepsy attending a UK epilepsy clinic reported 38% of patients claiming to have been burned at some time during a seizure compared to 7% recalling being burned at other times unrelated to seizures.[16] The most common type of burn injury was scalding from hot water and other fluids followed by contact or radiation burns from open fires or other heating appliances such as domestic radiators. Despite the relative frequency of burn injuries among people with epilepsy, it is apparent that patients recall very little advice on the specific risk of burn injuries occurring during a seizure and potential strategies for reducing that risk. Of the total cohort, only seven patients recalled ever being given advice about precautions to avoid burns injuries; of these, two were given the advice after they had already presented with burn injuries. This was significantly less than other guidance for more well-known risks of epilepsy, such as driving, operating machinery, or swimming.

A study based on 111 admissions into a UK Burns Unit revealed that the vast majority of burn injuries occur within a domestic as opposed to industrial setting. Of these, the most common were scald injuries resulting from cooking with boiling water, oil, or other fats or consumption of hot drinks. In addition, contact injuries were common, especially those caused by contact with radiators or hot stoves.[17] There is little evidence to suggest that presence of ID impacts upon the risk of sustaining a burn injury for people with epilepsy. A United States (US) study of patients attending an epilepsy clinic considered risk factors for burn injuries for patients with epilepsy. Interestingly, in logistical regression analysis, three significant variables were found to usefully predict risk of burn injuries, namely, number of seizures, presence of a neurological deficit, and gender. Neurological deficit was described as that which "demonstrably resulted in significant functional impairment." Developmental delay was however found to be a protective factor. This is presumably because in many cases, care arrangements are such that these patients are prevented from participating in, or at least being supervised in, those activities, such as cooking, most likely to result in burn injuries.[18] This is of interest, since an Australian study of the epidemiology of injuries among all patients with ID found that they were more likely to present to hospital with burn injuries than is the general population (5.3% compared with 1.3%), although this finding was not statistically significant.[19] It is likely that the epidemiology of burn injuries among those with ID will be distinct from the population as a whole, with a greater preponderance of burn injuries occurring during bathing or showering rather than during cooking and other domestic activities, primarily due to the lower likelihood of patients engaging in these activities or at least doing so unsupervised.[20] In one retrospective review based in the UK, of 18 patients presenting with serious burn injuries sustained during bathing or showering, four were people with ID.[21]

As with the population with epilepsy as a whole, precautions can and should be taken to prevent burn injuries occurring to patients with intellectual disability and coexisting epilepsy. The majority of burn injuries occur in a domestic setting, so simple precautions, such as the fitting of guards around fires, radiators, and cookers should be introduced. As discussed above, patients with ID may be less likely to engage in activities such as cooking, but if they do, those with coexisting epilepsy should be supervised at all times. Small measures, such as placing pans to the rear of the hob, ensuring saucepan handles do not overhang, and where possible, using microwave ovens and insulated kettles, should all be promoted. In addition, the fitting of thermostats to regulate water temperature in baths and showers and the adoption of shower curtains rather than solid cubicles should be considered to prevent burn injuries occurring during seizures.[22]

Drownings

Although in absolute terms deaths and injuries from drowning are infrequent for patients with epilepsy, they still represent a significant excess cause of death and hospital admission when compared with the population as a whole.[23] The pattern of drowning incidents is also distinct, since for most cases involving patients with epilepsy the drowning occurs in the bath as a result of a seizure, although other drownings during leisure activities such as swimming and sailing also occur and represent an excess risk. One retrospective cohort study based in Washington State calculated that a child with epilepsy was 96 times more likely to drown in the bath than a child without epilepsy and 23 times more likely to drown in a swimming pool.[24]

It is clear that this excess remains for patients with coexisting ID and that, in addition, ID itself is associated with increased drowning risk.[25] A 15-year observational study based in California[26] followed a cohort of over 200,000 people with ID to compare causes of death for those with and without epilepsy. It should be noted that those with the most severe forms of ID were excluded in order to minimize the possibility of confounding the risk of drowning due specifically to epilepsy with other factors associated with the severity of ID. Over this time period the authors reported 406 deaths for those patients with coexisting epilepsy, and of these 25 were due to drowning. This represented a 13-fold increased standardized mortality ratio compared to those people with ID but without epilepsy. The impact of excluding those with the severest forms of disability to avoid confounding on these results is open to conjecture, as the impact may be bidirectional. While for example they may have been at increased risk of drowning, increased care and supervision arrangements may have dictated that such risks were confined and that consequently the inclusion of the most severely disabled people within the cohort may have reduced the overall risk relative to the population without epilepsy.

Clearly drowning, particularly drowning occurring in the bath, is potentially avoidable. Within the UK, the National Institute of Clinical Excellence guidelines on this issue state that patients with coexisting ID and epilepsy should have a risk assessment that includes bathing provision.[27] The option of showering rather than bathing should be considered, although the risks of scalding resulting from seizures occurring during showering, as discussed above, should also be considered.[22] It has been shown that if children with epilepsy are supervised, they are at no greater risk of drowning than the general population.[28] Guidelines recommended for patients with epilepsy in general are also appropriate for those with coexisting ID.[29] These are that individuals should swim inside a pool rather than the sea, lake, or river, and one—to-one supervision by a responsible adult capable of reacting appropriately to any incidents that occur should be mandatory.

Fractures

It is well documented that the rate of fractures for people with epilepsy is higher than for the population as a whole.[30] While this is partly due to falls occurring during seizures, other mechanisms also exist. In particular, attention has focused on the impact of anticonvulsants on bone mineral density and the development of osteoporosis. In addition, a further impact may be the sedatory effects of anticonvulsants, which may increase the risk of falls.[31]

Patients with ID and coexisting epilepsy share the increased risk of fractures. Jancar and Jancar reported an incident fracture rate of 26% for patients with ID and with epilepsy compared with 15% in those without.[32] Of 68 fractures occurring in those patients with epilepsy, 17 (25%) occurred as a result of a seizure. In the UK, the admission rate for fractures to accident and emergency units was almost three times greater for patients with ID and with coexisting epilepsy compared with those without.[6]

A study based in the United States in a long-term care institution revealed an odds ratio for fracture of 1.9 for patients with epilepsy compared to those without.[33] Interestingly, the same study found no association between risk of fracture and severity of ID, although this may be due to the bidirectional nature of the relationship in that while severity of ID is associated with increased frequency of seizures, it is also associated with reduced mobility.

One case control study considering nontraumatic appendicular fractures among an institutionalized population reported an annual prevalence rate of 7.3%, sevenfold that expected in the general population.[34] There was an increased risk in those patients who were prescribed antiepileptic medication. Of cases who had a history of fracture, 83% were prescribed antiepileptic medication compared with 52% of controls. A South African based case-control study of patients with cerebral palsy also demonstrated a significant association between use of antiepileptic medication and number of fractures occurring.[35]

In the prospective observational Norwegian study by Nakken and colleagues[15] (see above) based on an observed cohort of 62 patients, nine fractures resulted from a total of 2,714 seizure-related falls over a 13-month period. Of these five were considered to be serious: two fractured legs, one mandibular fracture, one fractured neck of the femur, and one fractured skull.

In addition to the likelihood of fractures resulting from falls occurring during seizure, it is well documented that anticonvulsants are associated with low bone mineral density[36] and that duration of exposure to anticonvulsants is an important factor.[37]

Several potential mechanisms have been suggested to explain this association, including failure to synthesize or absorb vitamin D, calcium, vitamin K, and phosphorus.[38] Phenytoin, primidone, and phenobarbitone have all been shown to lead to osteomalacia.[39]

The prevalence of low bone mineral density and osteoporosis is significantly exceeded in patients with ID in general.[40,41] The extent of this, however, may be exaggerated, as many of the studies supporting this finding were conducted within institutions, and the two suggested mechanisms -- osteopenia and osteomalacia -- are associated with institutionalization. Osteopenia can occur as a result of immobility, which may be due to motor problems associated with the ID, which may also be increased due to institutional regimens. Osteomalacia is the softening of bone mass resulting from deficiency or inadequate metabolism of vitamin D. In institutionalized patients this may be due to insufficient exposure to sunlight. In addition, there is evidence of other medication for psychiatric and behavior disorders impacting on bone loss.

A further factor which should be noted is that risk of falls and fracture are predicted by the presence of generalized seizure,[42,43] and despite potential problems with diagnosis of seizure type it has been shown that patients with ID have an increased likelihood of generalized seizures compared with patients with epilepsy as a whole.[44,45]

To summarize, patients with ID and epilepsy may be have an inflated risk of fracture due to factors associated with both individual conditions. For all patients on anticonvulsants, osteoporosis should be considered as a potential comorbidity. Monitoring of bone density should be considered, and osteoporosis in these patients should be minimized by ensuring adequate nutrition, including supplements to provide optimal levels of calcium and vitamin D. Simple measures such as increasing exposure to sunlight for institutionalized patients might prove simple to implement and effective.

Head and Soft Tissue Injuries

Soft tissue injuries, particularly head injuries, have been shown to be the most common among patients with epilepsy and represent an excess compared with the general population.[46] Clearly this excess is largely explained by the impact of seizures themselves. Within a population of 255 residential patients with chronic long-term epilepsy studied over a one-month period, there were a total of 27,934 seizures, of which 45% resulted in falls. These led to 766 head injuries that were considered to be significant; of these, 422 (55%) were treated with a simple dressing and 341 (44%) required suturing . Two head injuries were accompanied with severe hemorrhage (one extradural and one subdural). A further injury resulted in a fractured skull.[47]

For patients with ID and coexisting epilepsy, this excess seems to remain. A UK study has reported that the admission rate to accident and emergency units for soft tissue injury following trauma was significantly increased for ID patients with coexisting epilepsy compared with those without.[6]

It is clear that certain characteristics of the type of epilepsy affecting those with ID predict increased incidence of falls, as previously discussed in relation to fractures. However, it should also be considered that while the incidence of soft tissue injuries related to fractures is relatively high, the incidence of injuries deemed to be serious is comparatively low.[46]

Mortality and Sudden Unexpected Death for People With Epilepsy

The risk of sudden unexpected death for people with epilepsy (SUDEP) is known to occur in excess. In a review article, Ficker reported a range of between 2% and 17% for the proportion of deaths among the population with epilepsy for which SUDEP was the cause.[48] For a diagnosis of SUDEP the following criteria apply:

1. The person must be known to have had epilepsy
2. The event can be witnessed or unwitnessed
3. Any deaths resulting from drowning or trauma are excluded
4. Any deaths resulting from status epilepticus are excluded
5. Evidence of a seizure does not need to be present
6. No toxicological or anatomical cause should be revealed during postmortem

There is evidence that SUDEP has been underreported and that the rate of reporting may vary by demographic and other factors. It is possible, for example, that postmortems are performed more frequently on the young and that in older people, evidence of disease such as arteriosclerosis may lead to a misdiagnosis of the cause of death.

Due to the complex nature and risk factors associated with epilepsy and ID it is difficult to disentangle the exact nature of the risk of SUDEP. Certain risk factors such as younger age, increased prevalence of generalized seizures, history of refractory epilepsy, and poorer control are factors likely to be associated with patients with ID and coexisting epilepsy. However, other factors may be protective. For example, patients within institutions or within formal care arrangements may have greater compliance with anticonvulsive medication.

There is conflicting evidence as to the impact of SUDEP among people with ID. A study based on the General Practice Research Database (GPRD) in the UK showed a modest increase in risk of SUDEP for patients with ID, but this was not statistically significant.[49] Similarly, a coroner-based study in Australia failed to show any increased risk of SUDEP for people with ID.[50]

An institution-based study in the US identified a rate of SUDEP for patients with ID as 20%. A description of risk factors for this population revealed similar findings to those of the population with epilepsy in general, namely, the number of antiepileptic drugs prescribed and the number of seizures recorded in the 12-month period prior to the death.[51]

A prospective US study showed a significant association between SUDEP and the presence of ID, which remained after controlling for the increased number of seizures occurring in the ID cohort. This study also proposes a potential mechanism to explain this increased risk based upon a combination of postictal apnea due to prolonged postictal encephalopathy,[26] which may decrease postictal respiratory drive. Furthermore, the neurological abnormalities often associated with mental retardation may preclude movement and righting reflexes if the patient is prone or supine following a generalized tonic-clonic seizure. For both of these reasons, mentally retarded patients may be more susceptible to the postictal central apnea and positional asphyxia that may cause SUDEP.

Use of Nonpsychiatric Hospital Services

In addition to the effect upon the well-being and quality of life of the individual patient, the physical health problems associated with epilepsy in the ID population impact upon the provision of health care services. Predictably ID is associated with increased inpatient utilization relative to the general population.[52]

A UK study based in South Wales demonstrated that this population are excess users of acute nonpsychiatric inpatient services. Naturally there is excess use within the neurology and general medical departments, as these are the specialties likely to be involved in the management of epilepsy. Excess use is also apparent within the trauma and orthopedic specialties, presumably reflecting the increased risk of trauma and fracture described above.

Other increased usage may reflect the association of epilepsy and severity of ID. Excesses in oral surgery may indicate the need for increased use of general anesthesia in this population, although the risk of dental injuries occurring during seizure has also been reported.[15]

Outpatient activity was increased, especially in those departments primarily responsible for the management of epilepsy, such as neurology, and for the treatment of soft tissue injuries and fractures in trauma and orthopedics. In addition, there is excess usage of mental handicap outpatient services, reflecting the increased severity of ID for those patients with coexisting epilepsy.

An interesting issue raised by the above study is the confounding impact of institutionalized care on health service utilization. The association of severity of disability with the presence of epilepsy inevitably leads to a higher prevalence of epilepsy among patients within institutions than among those resident in the community. It is possible that staff within the institution, particularly those with medical training, may provide an acute medical role. As such, the threshold of severity for seizures and any resulting injures, for accessing accident and emergency services, may be higher within institutions than in the community. Other studies have demonstrated reduced admission rates for institutionalized patients in general despite their perceived greater health needs.

Conclusion

As with many other areas concerning people with ID and epilepsy, the available specific information is sparse. There is comparatively little research concerning this population directly; instead, much must be extrapolated from the general population with epilepsy. Frequently the impact of ID is implied only as a risk factor or protective factor identified by statistical analysis. Clearly, however, there are certain differences that need to be observed. The increased risk of osteoporosis in the ID population increases the need for additional attention in preventing the risk of fracture in terms of providing supplements and possibly in determining appropriate pharmacology, both as antiepileptic medications and also other medications prescribed for other morbidities associated with the underlying ID. Supervision of bathing and showering is essential to prevent both burns and drowning. Simple measures, as outlined above, should be introduced. However, it is also necessary to remember that although injuries are excess in the population with ID and epilepsy, serious injury is still comparatively rare. It is therefore important to balance sensible precautions with the needs of the individual to live as full and independent a life as possible.

References

1. Kerr MP, Bowley C. (2000) Epilepsy and intellectual disability. J Intellect Disabil Res 44: 529–43.
2. Goodridge DM, Shorvon SD. (1983) Epileptic seizures in a population of 6000. I. Demography, diagnosis and classification, and role of the hospital services. BMJ 287: 641–4.
3. Richardson SA, Koller H, Katz M, et al. (1981). A functional classification of a seizures and its distribution in a mentally retarded population. Am J Ment Defic 85: 457–66.
4. Pueschel, SM, Rynders JE. (1982) Down syndrome:advances in biomedicine and the behavioral sciences. Cambridge, MA, USA: Ware Press, 169–225.
5. Aicardi J. (1994) Epilepsy as a presenting manifestation of brain tumors and of other selected brain disorders. In: Aicardi J (ed.). Epilepsy in children (The international review of child neurology), 2nd ed. New York: Raven Press, 350–1.
6. Morgan CL, Baxter HA, Kerr MP (2003) Prevalence of epilepsy and associated health service utilization and mortality among patients with intellectual disability. Am J Ment Retard 108: 293–300.
7. Patja K, Molsa P, Ivanainen M. (2001) Cause-specific mortality of people with intellectual disability in a population-based, 35-year follow-up study. J Intellect Disabil Res 45: 30–40.
8. Holland AJ. (2000) Ageing and mental retardation. Br J Psych 76: 26–31.
9. Strauss D, Eyman RK. (1996) Mortality of people with mental retardation in California with and without Down syndrome, 1986–1991. Am J Ment Retard 6(100): 643–53.
10. Wirrel EC. (2006) Epilepsy related injuries. Epilepsia 47(Suppl 1): 79–86.
11. Buck D, Baker GA, Jacoby A, et al. (1997). Patients' experiences of injury as a result of epilepsy. Epilepsia 38: 439–44.
12. Lawn ND, Bamlet WR, Radhakrishnan K, et al. (2004) Injuries due to seizures in persons with epilepsy: A population-based study. Neurology 63: 1565–70.
13. Beghi E, Cornaggia C. (2002) Morbidity and accidents in patients with epilepsy: Results of a European cohort study. Epilepsia 43: 1076–83.
14. Sherrard J, Tonge BJ, Ozanne-Smith J. (2002) Injury risk in young people with intellectual disability J Intellect Disabil Res 46: 6–10.
15. Nakken KO, Lossius R. (1993) Seizure related injuries in multihandicapped patients with therapy resistant epilepsy. Epilepsia 34: 836–40.
16. Hampton KK, Peatfield RC, Pullar T, et al. (1998) Burns because of epilepsy. BMJ 296: 1659–60.
17. Josty JC, Narayanan V, Dickson WA. (2000) Burns in patients with epilepsy: Changes in epidemiology and implications for burn treatment and prevention. Epilepsia 41: 453–6.
18. Spitz MC, Towbin JA, Shantz D, et al. (1994) Risk factors for burns as a consequence of seizures in persons with epilepsy. Epilepsia 35: 764–7.
19. Sherrard J, Tonge BJ, Ozanne-Smith J. (2001) Injury in young people with intellectual disability: Descriptive epidemiology. Injury Prev 7: 56–61.
20. Backstein R, Peters W, Neligan P. (1993). Burns in the disabled. Burns 19: 192–7.

21. Cerovac S, Roberts AH. (2000) Burns sustained by hot bath and shower water. Burns 26: 251–9.
22. Unglaub F, Woodruff S, Demir E, et al. (2005) Patients with epilepsy: A high-risk population prone to severe burns as a consequence of seizures while showering. J Burn Care Rehabil 26: 526–8.
23. Ryan CA, Dowling G. (1993) Drowning deaths in people with epilepsy. CMAJ 148: 781–4.
24. Diekema DS, Quan L, Holt VL. (1993) Epilepsy as a risk factor for submersion injury in children. Pediatrics 91: 612–6.
25. Kemp AM, Sibert JR. (1993) Epilepsy in children and the risk of drowning. Arch Dis Child 69: 684–5.
26. Day SM, Wu YW, Strauss DJ, et al. (2005) Causes of death in remote symptomatic epilepsy. Neurology 65: 216–22.
27. Stokes T. Shaw EJ, Juarez-Garcia A, et al. (2004). Clinical Guidelines and Evidence Review for the Epilepsies: diagnosis and management in adults and children in primary and secondary care. London: Royal College of General Practitioners.
28. Kemp AM, Sibert JR. (1993). Epilepsy in children and the risk of drowning. Arch Dis Child 68: 684–5.
29. Besag FMC. (2001) Tonic seizures are a particular risk factor for drowning in people with epilepsy. BMJ 322: 975–6.
30. Souverein PC, Webb DJ, Petri H, et al. (2005). Incidence of fractures among epilepsy patients: A population-based retrospective cohort study in the General Practice Research Database. Epilepsia 46: 304–10.
31. Souverein PC, Webb DJ, Weil JG, et al. (2006) Use of antiepileptic drugs and risk of fractures: Case-control study among patients with epilepsy. Neurology 66: 1318–24.
32. Jancar J, Jancar MP. (1998). Age-related fractures in people with intellectual disability and epilepsy. J Intellect Disabil Res. 42: 429–33.
33. Lohiya GS, Crinella FM, Tan-Figueroa L, et al. (1999). Fracture epidemiology and control in a developmental center. West J Med 170: 203–9.
34. Ryder KM, Williams J, Womack C, et al. (2003) Appendicular fractures: A significant problem among institutionalized adults with developmental disabilities. Am J Ment Retard 108: 340–6.
35. Bischof F, Basu D, Pettifor JM. (2002) Pathological long-bone fractures in residents with cerebral palsy in a long-term care facility in South Africa. Dev Med Child Neurol 44: 119–22.
36. Kinjo M, Setoguchi S, Schneeweiss S, et al. (2005) Bone mineral density in subjects using central nervous system-active medications. Am J Med 118: 1414.
37. Tolman KG, Jubiz W, Sannella JJ, et al. (1975) Osteomalacia associated with anticonvulsant drug therapy in mentally retarded children. Pediatrics 56: 45–50.
38. Imran AI, Schuh L, Barley GL, et al. (2004) Antiepileptic durgs and reduced bone mineral density. Epilepsy Behav 5: 296–300.
39. Winnacker JL, Yeager H, Saunders JA, et al. (1977). Rickets in children receiving anticonvulsant drugs: Biochemical and hormonal markers. Am J Dis Child 131: 286–90.
40. Schmidt EV, Byars JR, Flamuth DH, et al. (2004) Prevalence of low bone–mineral density among mentally retarded and developmentally disabled residents in intermediate care. Consult Pharm 19:45–51.
41. Lohiya GS, Tan-Figueroa L, Iannucci A. (2004) Identification of low bone mass in a developmental center: Finger bone mineral density measurement in 562 residents. J Am Med Dir Assoc 5: 371–6.
42. Persson HB Alberts KA, Farahmand BY, et al. (2002) Risk of extremity fractures in adult outpatients with epilepsy. Epilepsia 43: 768–72.
43. Neufeld MY, Vishne T, Chistik V, et al. (1999) Life-long history of injuries related to seizures. Epilepsy Res 34: 123–7.
44. Shepherd C, Hosking G. (1989) Epilepsy in school children with intellectual impairments in Sheffield: The size and nature of the problem and the implications for service provision. J Ment Defic Res 33: 511–4.

45. Mariani E, Ferini-Strambi L, Sala M, et al. (1993) Epilepsy in institutionalized patients with encephalopathy: Clinical aspects and nosological considerations. Am J Ment Retard 98 (Supp l): 27–33.
46. Lawn ND, Bamlet WR, Radhakrishnan K, et al. (2004) Injuries due to seizures in persons with epilepsy: A population-based study. Neurology 63: 1565–70.
47. Russell-Jones DL, Shorvon SD. (1989) The frequency and consequences of head injury in epileptic seizures. J Neurol Neurosurg Psychiat 52: 659–62.
48. Ficker D. (2000) Sudden unexplained death and injury in epilepsy. Epilepsia 41(Suppl 2): S7–12. Review.
49. Derby LE, Tennis P, Jick H. (1996) Sudden unexplained death among subjects with refractory epilepsy. Epilepsia 37: 931–5.
50. Opeskin K, Berkovic SF. (2003) Risk factors for sudden unexpected death in epilepsy: A controlled prospective study based on coroners cases. Seizure 12: 456–64.
51. McKee JR, Bodfish JW. (2000) Sudden unexpected death in epilepsy in adults with mental retardation. Am J Ment Retard 105: 229–35.
52. Walsh KK, Kastner T, Criscione T. (1997) Characteristics of hospitalizations for people with developmental disabilities: Utilization, costs and impact of care coordination. Am J Ment Retard 101: 505–20.

Chapter 12
Epilepsy and Cognition

M.L. Smith

Introduction

The effects of epilepsy are felt in multiple aspects of the person's life, including physical and mental health, cognitive function, educational achievements, vocational prospects, and family and peer relations.[1]. Cognition, which includes processes such as intelligent thinking, perceiving, remembering, reasoning, judging, expressing, and understanding, has an important role in the inception, evolution, and manifestation of many of these other aspects of function recognized to be compromised in people with epilepsy. Most cases of epilepsy have their onset in childhood, and thus seizure onset commonly occurs at a time that is essential to the development of basic cognitive, behavioral, and social skills that are crucial for long-term educational, vocational, and interpersonal adaptation.[2-4]. Therefore, an understanding of the cognitive deficits associated with epilepsy and of their predisposing factors is essential for appreciating the full impact of epilepsy.

Deficits in cognition are identified by people with epilepsy and their families as a significant comorbidity. For example, in a study by Arunkumar and colleagues,[5] parents of 80 children and adolescents with epilepsy were asked to list in order of importance their concerns about living with or caring for their children with epilepsy; children who were old enough to be interviewed were asked to express (independently of their parents) their own concerns about having epilepsy. For both parents and children, the second most common item identified was that of the cognitive effects of epilepsy. Their worries included learning disabilities, academic difficulties, poor attention and concentration, and impoverished memory. In terms of impact, these issues are not specific to children; in a survey by the International Bureau of Epilepsy, 44% of patients with epilepsy complained of difficulty learning, and 45% of slowness in thinking.[6] It has also been demonstrated that cognitive function is a significant predictor of self-evaluation of quality of life among adults with epilepsy.[7]

Although the majority of people with epilepsy have normal intelligence, the distribution of Intelligent Quotient (IQ) scores is skewed toward lower values.[8-11] A study by Smith and colleagues[12] of 51 children with medically refractory epilepsy illustrated the wide range of cognitive functioning within this group. The

V.P. Prasher, M.P. Kerr (eds.) *Epilepsy and Intellectual Disabilities*,
DOI: 10.1007/978-1-84800-259-3_12, © Springer Science+Business Media, LLC 2008

mean IQ was 84 (in the Low Average range, just over one standard deviation below the population mean of 100). The spread of IQ scores was considerable, spanning the Intellectually Deficient range (<1st percentile) to the Very Superior range (>99th percentile). In a study designed to document the occurrence of disabilities in an unselected population sample of children in Finland, 4–15 years of age, Sillanpaa[13] reported that the prevalence of epilepsy in the study population was 0.68%. Among the children with epilepsy, neurological deficit was found in 39.9%, the most frequent neurological impairments being intellectual disabilities (ID) (31.4%), speech disorders (27.5%), and specific learning disorders (23.1%). Even in individuals with normal intelligence, reports of deficits in specific aspects of neuropsychological functioning are common, particularly in the areas of attention and concentration, memory, executive function, and academic achievement. . Each of these areas will be briefly reviewed, as will a specific subset of developmental epilepsy syndromes that have a devastating effect on cognitive development. In addition, the effects of antiepileptic medications, and the potential effects of seizure-related variables on cognition, will be addressed.

Attention and Concentration

Selective attention, concentration, and the ability to sustain one's focus are important for the efficient completion of many tasks in life. . Deficits in attention are relatively common in people with epilepsy and can have far reaching consequences because attentional processes can also affect other aspects of cognition such as memory, language, and problem solving.[14] Attentional deficits may be distinguished from generalized cognitive impairment. Depressed performance on tests of attention has been documented even in patients with normal IQ.[15–16] Weaknesses in attentional processing were found to be disproportionate to the level of IQ in a sample of patients with ID.[17]

Kalviainen and colleagues[18] found that 30% of newly diagnosed adults with untreated seizures and no brain lesion had deficits in sustained attention and mental flexibility, even though attention span, speed of tracking, and psychomotor speed were intact. Patients with complex partial seizures are impaired on tasks requiring sustained concentration.[19] Children with epilepsy have been shown to have slowed reaction time and impairments in selective and sustained attention.[16,20–21] Not surprisingly, attentional deficits have been associated with educational problems. Teachers of children with epilepsy have reported difficulties in attention, concentration, and information processing, and they perceive these children as being less alert than their classmates.[22]

An increased risk for attention deficit hyperactivity disorder (ADHD) in children with epilepsy has been reported in many studies,[23] with estimates ranging from 17% to 58%. . Prevalence of ADHD does not appear to vary by seizure type or between localization-related versus generalized epilepsies.[23] Children with epilepsy and ADHD differ from other samples of children with ADHD by the higher proportion of children with ADHD predominantly inattentive type and by an equal male:female ratio.[24]

There are potentially important consequences for cognition of the coexistence of ADHD and epilepsy. A comparison of groups of children with complex partial seizures with and without ADHD, children with ADHD alone, and healthy controls demonstrated that those with seizures have significant difficulty with sustained attention and maintenance of consistency of responding over time regardless of diagnosis of ADHD. However, impairments on attention tasks were greatest in the combined seizure plus ADHD group.[25]

There is little consensus on the seizure variables that contribute to the behavioral and cognitive aspects of inattention in epilepsy.[23] There are studies that show that seizure type, seizure history, and drug therapy do not predict performance on tests of reaction time and attention,[20,26,27] whereas Aldenkamp and colleagues[28] found that patients with frequent epileptiform discharges and a history of drug polytherapy were most impaired on tests of vigilance and reaction time. It has been suggested that abnormal cortical or subcortical substrates underlie the attentional deficits, irrespective of seizure type.

Memory

Memory problems are among the most common complaints of people with epilepsy. Thompson and Corcoran[29] conducted a survey of 760 people with epilepsy and asked about the frequency of everyday memory failures, such as forgetting where things have been put, of losing things, going back to check if one had done something that one had intended to do, and being unable to say a word, although the word was known and "on the tip of one's tongue." The people with epilepsy not only endorsed a higher frequency of such events, but also rated the nuisance arising from such memory failures as higher than did people without epilepsy. Of further interest was the finding that relatives rated the frequency of forgetting among their family members with epilepsy as higher than did the persons themselves, suggesting that people with epilepsy may forget how often they do forget.

Memory deficits are most consistently observed in patients with epileptogenic foci involving the mesial temporal lobe. In most instances, the impairments seen with unilateral foci are material-specific in nature, as related to the hemisphere of the lesion (for reviews see Jones-Gotman and Smith[30]; Smith and Bigel.[31]. Studies have shown that, in patients with speech representation in the left hemisphere, epilepsy involving the mesial left temporal structures typically results in impairments on tasks of verbal learning and verbal memory. These individuals have difficulty with material presented in stories or text, with real or nonsense words, verbal paired-associate learning, recall of the names of actual or pictured objects, and to learning and remembering names of unfamiliar people. Right temporal lobe epilepsy has been associated with impaired performance on tasks in which the stimuli are difficult to verbalize, such as complex geometric designs, on learning across trials of lists of designs, and on the recognition of faces, recurring nonsense figures, and unfamiliar tonal melodies.[30,31] The specificity between side of focus and type of material is not always found, and more recently it has been argued that the memory requirements of the task, specifically learning over several trials, may be the critical feature in determining the specificity of a lesion effect.[32-33]

Bilateral damage to the mesial temporal lobe structures can result in a severe global amnesia.[34] In patients with bilateral epileptogenic foci, the memory impairments are generalized in nature, involving all modalities of input and both verbal and nonverbal memoranda. However, despite having strikingly impaired memories, most patients with bitemporal epilepsy are not amnesic.[30,35]

The study of memory in epilepsy has also examined remote and autobiographical memory. It has been shown that people with temporal lobe epilepsy have difficulty retrieving information based on past experiences as well as information based on recent events or new learning.[36-39] Despite these deficits in the personal episodic realm (specific events), memory for personal semantic information (facts about oneself) can remain intact.[37,39] These remote memory deficits have been demonstrated in both left and right temporal lobe epilepsy, although in some instances they may be related to the hemisphere of seizure onset. For example, right but not left temporal lobe foci have been associated with impairments in familiarity judgements for famous faces, but foci in either temporal lobe can result in impairments in naming such faces or in providing information about famous people.[39]

Like adults, children with temporal lobe epilepsy experience memory deficits. For children with medically controlled seizures, findings with respect to material-specific effects have been equivocal, with some studies demonstrating verbal memory deficits in conjunction with left temporal foci, and spatial memory deficits in conjunction with right temporal foci[40-43] and others not showing this pattern of specificity.[44-45] Children with intractable seizures arising from the temporal lobe typically have memory disorders that have not been described as material-specific.[46-51] This difference between adults and children may have to do with age of seizure onset or duration of epilepsy.

Executive Functions

A set of complex cognitive processes have been grouped under the construct "executive functions," or those skills required to maintain an appropriate problem-solving set for the attainment of future goals. Among patients with epilepsy, as with other types of neurological compromise, impairments of executive function have been associated with frontal-lobe abnormality. In a comparison of adults with frontal lobe epilepsy and temporal lobe epilepsy, the former were found to have inferior performance on tests of memory span, visual motor speed, selective attention, visual perceptual speed, response inhibition, verbal fluency, concept formation, planning, and motor coordination.[52] Factor analysis of the results identified four frontal subfunctions: speed/attention, response maintenance and inhibition, motor coordination, and short-term memory. Both frontal and temporal lobe epilepsy were associated with deficits in the short-term memory and speed/attention domains, whereas only patients with frontal-lobe seizures were characterized by impairments in the motor coordination and/or response inhibition domains. In patients with epileptogenic foci in the frontal lobes, impairments have not been found to be related to the laterality of the focus, or to the site of localization within the frontal lobe.[52-54]

Case studies of children have described the onset of frontal-lobe seizures accompanied by behavioral, cognitive, and motor impairments that were reversed when seizure control was obtained with pharmacotherapy.[55,56] Group studies have demonstrated that children with frontal lobe epilepsy have deficits in attention, planning, categorization, organization, memory, impulse control, verbal fluency, comprehension, and motor coordination.[57-62] Prevost and colleagues[63] found a significant incidence of attention deficits, behavior problems, and learning disabilities in children with nonlesional frontal lobe epilepsy. In these group studies, the appearance of abnormalities appears to be independent of seizure control.

In children with medically controlled epilepsy, some differences have been documented between the effects of frontal and temporal lobe seizures. Those with frontal lobe seizures perform more poorly on motor coordination, verbal fluency, and planning ability, whereas children with temporal lobe seizures perform more poorly on tests of verbal memory.[58,59,61] In children with intractable epilepsy, differences do not appear to be as prevalent, and these two groups have been shown to have similar performance on tasks of verbal fluency, comprehension, attention, and verbal and visuospatial memory.[57,60]

Academic Function

Children with epilepsy are at risk for delays in academic skills and for specific learning disabilities in the core academic areas of reading, spelling, and arithmetic.[64-67] The nature of the learning difficulties is not limited to these traditional areas, and underachievement has been reported for all academic subjects.[68] Prevalence rates of learning problems reported in the literature have ranged from 5–70%.[69,70] While these problems may be especially prevalent in children with chronic seizures, there is a relatively high risk, even among those with relatively recent onset and with uncomplicated, well-controlled seizures.[71,72] A prospective study of childhood-onset epilepsy suggested that even in individuals who eventually became medication and seizure free, academic problems persisted into adulthood.[73]

There are large individual differences in the incidence, nature, and severity of the academic delays, and a constellation of factors has been identified as potential determinants. Seizure severity, seizure frequency, and side effects of antiepileptic drugs (AEDs) have been identified as contributors.[45,72,74] Child adaptive competency, (a variable that includes constructs such as degree of effort, behavior, learning, and mood) is related to achievement in both children with recent-onset and chronic epilepsy.[71,72]

The academic deficits can be differentiated from more generalized impairments in intelligence and cognition, although deficits in the latter such as in attention, motor fluency, alertness, speed of information processing, and memory, can contribute to the struggles of these children in learning in the school environment.[45,74] For example, in a narrative study of quality of life,[69] youth with intractable epilepsy reported that they frequently felt that they were physically or mentally unavailable to learn and, therefore, were unable to count on a continuous and integrated learning experience. Fatigue and problems with memory were identified as influences that compromised their performance at school. Furthermore, children with epilepsy may differ from children with learning disabilities arising from other etiologies, in terms of the underlying cognitive correlates; for example, children with epilepsy have slower reaction times on a variety of simple and complex auditory and visual reaction time tasks than do learning disabled children without epilepsy.[75]

Level of intelligence influences the likelihood of learning disability. In a population-based cohort of adults with childhood-onset epilepsy,[76] 76% had a history of learning disability. The occurrence of learning disability was closely linked to IQ. Half of the patients (51%) with learning disability had ID. Among those with IQs in the normal range or above, the prevalence was 57%, in the mentally near-normal (IQ=71–85) it was 67%, and in those with ID (IQ>71), all had learning disabilities by self-definition. Intellectual disabilities and subsequent learning disability were predicted by presence of cerebral palsy, onset of epilepsy before the age of six years, and poor early response to AEDs. Among intellectually normal or near-normal subjects, a symptomatic etiology of epilepsy was the only predictor of a learning disability. The degree of learning disability significantly affected medical, social, and educational long-term outcomes.

One approach to understanding the relationship between epilepsy and academic achievement might be in the comparison of epilepsy syndromes.[77] Children with idiopathic generalized or with localization-related epilepsy have been found to have a higher probability of mainstream schooling than those with symptomatic or cryptogenic generalized epilepsy or undetermined epilepsy syndromes.[78] Vanasse and colleagues[79] examined reading skills in children with temporal lobe epilepsy, frontal lobe epilepsy, or absence epilepsy. All groups were reading at levels approximately two years behind expectations. Children in the frontal lobe group, and to a lesser extent, those in the absence group, had deficits on tasks related to phonological processing, whereas those with temporal lobe epilepsy did not differ from controls. An epileptogenic focus in the frontal lobe apparently affects the phonological underpinnings of reading. This finding suggests that the syndrome approach may reveal a relationship between specific epileptogenic features and other component processes underlying the academic skills.

Other Cognitive Functions

In patients with foci in the left lateral temporal cortex, mild impairments have been documented in the areas of verbal perception,[80] object naming,[81] and language processing.[82] Impairments in span of attention or working memory have also been noted in patients with temporal neocortical epilepsy.[83] An association between impaired discourse ability and working memory has been found in patients with temporal lobe epilepsy.[84] Mild visual perceptual deficits have been reported in association with foci in the right temporal lobe.[85]

Intractable Epilepsy Syndromes of Childhood

Intractable epilepsy syndromes of childhood onset are associated with a high risk for cognitive impairment and frequently for global developmental delays. To illustrate this association, a brief review of four syndromes follows.

Infantile Spasms.

The syndrome of infantile spasms begins in the middle of the first year of life with the onset of characteristic flexor spasms.[86] Development of cognitive and motor function may be normal or abnormal prior to onset, and deterioration in development commonly, although not inevitably, accompanies the onset of seizures.[87] The developmental outcome is likely related to the underlying etiology; many of the symptomatic cases are seen in association with genetic disorders or cortical malformations that in themselves carry risk for generalized developmental delays.[88,89]

Lennox-Gastaut Syndrome.

Lennox-Gastaut syndrome is characterized by three features: multiple seizure types, slow spike and wave disturbance with bursts of fast rhythms on EEG, and psychological disturbances, including psychomotor delay, personality disorders, or both.[86,90] In some children with no identifiable etiology, psychomotor retardation may be evident before the onset of seizures, but the psychological abnormalities typically appear in conjunction with the first seizure or evolve shortly thereafter.[90] The level of IQ deteriorates progressively over time, either as a consequence of developmental arrest or loss of previously acquired skills. The vast majority of cases have marked ID, which may be most pronounced in children who previously had infantile spasms.[91]

Landau-Kleffner Syndrome

The syndrome of "acquired aphasia with convulsive disorder in children" was first described by Landau and Kleffner[92] in six children with normal early language development who suddenly developed aphasia in relation to an epileptic disorder. The language disturbance typically first involves verbal comprehension (classicly a verbal auditory agnosia) that may be mistaken for an acquired deafness. The usually gradual deterioration in verbal production follows the loss of comprehension, occurs together with it, or even precedes it. Several variables can influence the severity and the duration of the language disorder: frequency of the epileptic discharges in the language zones, the duration of the epileptic disorder, the spread of the epileptic discharges to the homologous contralateral cortex, and the efficacy of the AED therapy.[93,94]

Severe Myoclonic Epilepsy in Infancy

Severe myoclonic epilepsy in infancy typically has its onset in the middle of the first year of life and begins with tonic or tonic-clonic seizures, with later occurrence of myoclonic jerks, atypical absence seizures, and partial seizures. Development prior to the onset of seizures is usually normal, but later development is slow, behavioral problems are frequent, and motor skills become compromised. The cognitive impairments are usually generalized, and the behavioral features include hyperactivity, autistic traits, and impaired interpersonal relations.[95,96]

Antiepileptic Drugs

Antiepileptic drugs reduce the propensity for seizures by decreasing neuronal excitability or by enhancing inhibitory neurotransmission, and by these same mechanisms can produce cognitive side effects.[97,98] A number of physical side effects, such as sedation, somnolence, insomnia, or dizziness, may affect multiple aspects of cognition. Other effects may more directly impact specific aspects of cognition, such as psychomotor slowing, reduced vigilance, distractibility, language impairment, and memory impairment. These side effects can significantly impact on daily functions in multiple domains. It has been shown that there is a strong negative relationship between self-reported adverse effects of AEDs and perception of quality of life.[99]

Many reviews of side effects of AEDs distinguish between "traditional" and "newer" drugs.[100,101] The traditional category – drugs available prior to the 1990s – includes phenobarbital, phenytoin, valproate, primidone, ethosuximide, and carbamazepine. These drugs have been associated with clinically significant side effects.[98] Of these, phenobarbital has been most frequently associated with adverse cognitive and behavioral consequences, including attentional deficits, hyperactivity, decreased short-term memory, and conduct disturbances.[102] Phenytoin has been associated with declines in intellectual function.[103] These effects appear to be most pronounced in patients with more severe epilepsy, coexisting neurobehavioral disorders, and drug toxicity.[51] Many of the studies on these traditional AEDs have been confounded by methodological limitations,[104] and it is not always possible to disentangle potential side effects from effects due to ongoing seizures, preexisting disorders, or other factors.

Studies that have attempted to control for such confounds have not always found effects of AEDs. For example, Williams and colleagues[51] followed up with 37 children with newly diagnosed epilepsy for six months. A baseline assessment was conducted prior to the initiation of AED treatment, and performance was compared with a control group of children with newly diagnosed epilepsy. Children were treated with monotherapy, and blood serum levels were in the therapeutic range throughout the six-month follow-up period. At baseline, significant group differences were not present, although the children with epilepsy performed more poorly than the controls on all cognitive measures and were rated as having more problematic behavior. However, changes in performance over the six months did not differ between the children with epilepsy and the control group.

In healthy adult volunteers, in whom the effects of the drugs can be assessed without the confounds of seizures, neuropathology, genetic vulnerabilities, and psychosocial factors, the effects of the traditional AEDs have been modest and similar across carbamazepine, phenytoin, and valproate, whereas phenobarbital has a more adverse effect than the latter two. However, all of phenobarbital, phenytoin, valproate, and carbamazepine result in impairments of cognitive function and/or motor speed when compared with a no-drug control condition.[100,105] The newer AEDs, including gabapentin, levetiracetam, lamotrigine, oxcarazepine, and tiagabine, tend to be associated with fewer side effects than the traditional ones.[101,105] Topiramate has documented effects in both healthy controls and patients with epilepsy, adversely affecting concentration, processing speed, and aspects of verbal function, including intelligence, fluency, learning, and short-term memory.[106-109] The effects of topiramate are accentuated when administered at higher doses, with rapid titration, and in combination therapy.[98]

Many of these findings are based on trials and clinical experience with adults, and the results may not generalize to all ages. There may be some age-specific side effects of AEDs that can reduce cognitive efficiency, such as depression in adults and aggression and hyperactivity in children.[98] There is a pressing need for well-designed AED drug trials in both the elderly and in children. . The elderly may have different absorption and metabolic rates than younger adults, there are age-related physiological changes that influence the metabolism of AEDs, and the elderly tend to have a greater number of other medical conditions.[98,110] The effects of AEDs may be different in the developing than in the adult brain.[98,101] Long-term consequences of AEDs can be particularly devastating in children, as even modest cognitive impairments may have cumulative consequences if they affect learning and limit the acquisition of academic skills.[99] Children with ID may be more susceptible to cognitive loss after AED treatment.[111,112] Children with pre-existing behavior disorders such as attention deficit disorder may be more vulnerable to an exacerbation of behavioral difficulties.[111,112]

Other Influences on Cognition

A multitude of studies have addressed questions about the specific features of the seizure disorder in their implications for the appearance and severity of cognitive deficits. Some of these features have been covered in more depth (such as the localization and laterality of seizures) or have merely been touched on in the preceding sections. In this final section, a discussion of epileptiform discharges, duration of epilepsy, frequency of seizures, and age is presented.

Attention, language, and memory may be disrupted by subclinical epileptiform discharges, a phenomenon known as transient cognitive impairment.[113] Transient cognitive impairment apparently results from the effects of these subclinical discharges on brain function, rather than from the underlying brain pathology.[114]

Two interrelated variables have received considerable attention for their impact on cognitive function: duration of epilepsy and age of seizure onset. Hermann and colleagues[115] found an association between age at seizure onset, neuropsychological function, and brain structure. Adults with onset of temporal lobe epilepsy earlier in childhood (mean of 7.8 years) had a more diffuse pattern of cognitive deficits (i.e., greater degree of impairment and evident across a greater number of cognitive domains), and showed more magnetic resonance imaging structural abnormalities (particularly a reduction in white matter volume) that extended into the extratemporal regions, beyond the site of epileptogenic focus, than did adults with later-onset temporal lobe epilepsy (mean of 23.3 years). This study is important in that it demonstrated an association between age of onset, cognitive dysfunction, and extent of brain abnormality. The authors concluded that childhood-onset temporal lobe epilepsy is associated with an adverse neurodevelopmental impact on brain structure and cognition.

Thompson and Duncan[116] reported on 136 patients with a median duration of epilepsy of 35 years who had undergone cognitive testing on two occasions with a median retest interval of 13 years. They found decline in all areas assessed (intelligence, memory, naming, verbal fluency, and mental flexibility). This finding is consistent with earlier studies. For example, a review of longitudinal studies of intelligence in children with epilepsy identified several studies in which patients with a four-year or longer duration of seizures showed a decline in intelligence, suggesting the conclusion that seizures had a causative role in this decline.[117] Declines in intelligence over time have been reported among patients with poor seizure control, whereas patients who had experienced improvements in seizure control have shown gains in intellectual performance.[118–120] Among patients with temporal lobe epilepsy followed over a four-year interval, cognitive prognosis was poor for a subset (20–25%) characterized by chronicity of epilepsy, older age, lower intellectual ability at baseline, and more baseline abnormalities in quantitative magnetic resonance volumetrics.[121]

Other studies have failed to identify changes related to the duration of epilepsy or changes in seizure control.[122,123] In attempting to reconcile these differences across studies, it has been suggested that seizure frequency and type rather than duration may be of importance. For example, it has been found that the frequency of generalized tonic clonic seizures predicts decline in cognitive function among chronic epilepsy patients.[116,124] A history of status epilepticus has been associated with decline in memory.[116,124]

The majority of studies that have investigated age as a factor in cognitive impairment focused on age at seizure onset or duration. More recently, attention has been given to the elderly, a group at risk for developing epilepsy and for cognitive impairment associated with aging. . Elderly patients with focal epilepsy have been found to differ from demographically matched controls in diverse areas of cognition, including attention, perseveration, memory, construction, conceptualization, and verbal fluency.[125–127] Age of seizure onset and seizure duration were not associated with neurocognitive function,[125] but performance was related to AED polytherapy.[125–127] Seniors with epilepsy were found to have more pronounced deficits in aspects of executive function than older adults diagnosed with mild cognitive impairment.[126]

Conclusion

This review has identified the increased risk for impairment in multiple aspects of cognitive function in persons with epilepsy. The precise factors determining the appearance or severity of thee deficits are not completely understood. Nonetheless, individuals with epilepsy, families, social support networks, and health care providers need to be aware of these issues in order to understand the full impact of epilepsy. Proper and early identification is necessary to provide early developmental interventions, appropriate school programming, vocational counseling, supportive work settings, and a safe environment for promotion of independence across the life span.

References

1. Jalava M, Sillanpaa M, Camfield C, et al. (1997) Social adjustment and competence 35 years after onset of childhood epilepsy: A prospective controlled study. Epilepsia. 38: 708–715.
2. Hermann BP. (1982) Neuropsychological functioning and psychopathology in children with epilepsy. Epilepsia 23: 545–554.
3. Hermann BP, Black RB, Chhabria S. (1981) Behavioral problems and social competence in children with epilepsy. Epilepsia 22: 703–710.

4. Seidenberg M, Berent S. (1992) Childhood epilepsy and the role of psychology. Am Psychol 47: 1130–1133.
5. Arunkumar G, Wyllie E, Kotagal P, et al. (2000) Parent- and patient-validated content for pediatric epilepsy quality-of-life assessment. Epilepsia 41: 1474–1484.
6. Cognitive Function Survey. (2004) International Bureau for Epilepsy, www.ibe-epilepsy.org/whatsnewdet.asp.
7. Perrine K, Hermann BP, Meador KJ, et al. (1995) The relationship of neuropsychological functioning to quality of life in epilepsy. Arch Neurol. 52: 997–1003.
8. Bourgeois BF, Prensky AL, Palkes HS, et al. (1983) Intelligence in epilepsy: A prospective study in children. Ann Neurol 14: 438–444.
9. Ellenberg JH, Hirtz DG, Nelson KB. (1986) Do seizures in children cause intellectual deterioration? N Engl J Med 314: 1085–1088.
10. Sillanpaa M. (1990) Children with epilepsy as adults: Outcome after 30 years of follow-up. Acta Paediatr Scand Suppl 368: 1–78.
11. Tartar, RE. (1972) Intellectual and adaptive functioning in epilepsy. A review of 50 years of research. Dis Nerv Syst 33: 763–770.
12. Smith ML, Elliott IM, Lach L. (2002) Cognitive skills in children with intractable epilepsy: Comparison of surgical and non-surgical candidates. Epilepsia 43: 631–637.
13. Sillanpaa M. (1992) Epilepsy in children: Prevalence, disability, and handicap. Epilepsia 33: 444–449.
14. Kadis DS, Stollstorff M, Elliott I, et al. (2004) Cognitive and psychological predictors of everyday memory in children with intractable epilepsy. Epilepsy Behav 5: 37–43.
15. Smith DB, Craft BR, Collins J, et al. (1986) Behavioral characteristics of epilepsy patients compared with normal controls. Epilepsia. 27: 760–768.
16. Williams J, Griebel ML, Dykman RA. (1998) Neuropsychological patterns in pediatric epilepsy. Seizure 7: 223–228.
17. Forceville EJM, Dekker MJA, Aldenkamp AP, et al. (1992) Subtest profiles of the WISC-R and WAIS in mentally retarded patients with epilepsy. J Intellect Disabil Res. 36: 45–59.
18. Kalviainen R, Aikia M, Helkala EL, et al. (1992) Memory and attention in newly diagnosed epileptic seizure disorder. Seizure. 1: 255–262.
19. Stella F Maciel JA. (2003) Attentional disorders in patients with complex partial epilepsy. Arq Neuropsiquiatr. 61: 335–338.
20. Mitchell WG, Zhou Y, Chavez JM, et al. (1992) Reaction time, attention, and impulsivity in epilepsy. Pediatr Neurol. 8: 19–24.
21. Oostrom KJ, Schouten A, Kruitwagen CLJJ, et al. (2002) Attention deficits are not characteristic of schoolchildren with newly diagnosed idiopathic or cryptogenic epilepsy. Epilepsia. 43: 301–310.
22. Bennett-Levy J, Stores G. (1984) The nature of cognitive dysfunction in school-children with epilepsy. Acta Neurol Scand Suppl 99: 79–82.
23. Schubert R. (2005) Attention deficit disorder and epilepsy. Pediatr Neurol. 32: 1–10.
24. Dunn, DW, Austin, JK, Harezlak J, et al. (2003) ADHD and epilepsy in childhood. Dev Med Child Neurol. 45: 50–54.
25. Semrud-Clikeman M, Wical B. (1999) Components of attention in children with complex partial seizures with and without ADHD. Epilepsia. 40: 211–215.
26. Bailet LL, Turk WR. (2000) The impact of childhood epilepsy on neurocognitive and behavioral performance: A prospective longitudinal study. Epilepsia 41: 426–431.
27. McCarthy AM, Richman LC, Yarbrough D. (1995) Memory, attention and school problems in children with seizure disorders. Dev Neuropsychol. 11: 71–86.
28. Aldenkamp AP, Weber B, Overweg-Plandsoen WC, et al. (2005) Educational underachievement in children with epilepsy: A model to predict the effects of epilepsy on educational achievement. J Child Neurol 20: 175–180.
29. Thompson PJ, Corcoran 1R. (1992) Everyday memory failures in people with epilepsy. Epilepsia 33 (Suppl 6): S18–20.
30. Jones-Gotman M, Smith ML. (2006) Neuropsychological profiles. Adv Neurol. 97: 357–366.

31. Smith ML, Bigel MG. (2000) Temporal lobes and memory. In:. Cermak L (ed.). The handbook of neuropsychology, 2nd ed., Elsevier, Oxford.

32. Jones-Gotman M, Zatorre RJ, Olivier A, et al. (1997) Learning and retention of words and designs following excision from medial or lateral temporal-lobe structures. Neuropsychologia 35: 963–973.

33. Dade LA, Jones-Gotman M. (2001) Face learning and memory: The Twins Test. Neuropsychology. 15: 525–534.

34. Milner B. (2005) The medial temporal-lobe amnesic syndrome. Psychiatr Clin North Am 28: 599–611.

35. Guerreiro CA, Jones-Gotman M, Andermann F, et al. (2001) Severe amnesia in epilepsy: Causes, anatomopsychological considerations, and treatment. Epilepsy Behav 2: 224–246.

36. Lah S, Lee T, Grayson S, et al. (2006) Effects of temporal lobe epilepsy on retrograde memory. Epilepsia 47: 615–625.

37. Viskontas IV, McAndrews MP, Moscovitch M. (2000) Remote episodic memory deficits in patients with unilateral temporal lobe epilepsy and excisions. J Neurosci 20: 5853–5857.

38. Viskontas IV, McAndrews MP, Moscovitch M. (2002) Memory for famous people in patients with unilateral temporal lobe epilepsy and excisions. Neuropsychology 16: 472–480.

39. Voltzenlogel V, Despres O, Vignal JP, et al. (2006) Remote memory in temporal lobe epilepsy. Epilepsia 47: 1329–1336.

40. Beardsworth ED, Zaidel DW. (1994) Memory for faces in epileptic children before and after brain surgery. J Clin Exp Neuropsych 16: 589–596.

41. Cohen M. (1992) Auditory/verbal and visual/spatial memory in children with complex partial epilepsy of temporal lobe origin. Brain Cogn 20: 315–326.

42. Fedio, P, Mirsky A. (1969) Selective intellectual deficits in children with temporal lobe or centrencephalic epilepsy. Neuropsychologia 7: 287–300.

43. Jambaqué I, Dellatolas G, Dulac O, et al. (1993) Verbal and visual memory impairment in children with epilepsy. Neuropsychologia. 31: 1321–1327.

44. Hershey T, Craft S, Glauser TA, et al. (1998) Short-term and long-term memory in early temporal lobe dysfunction. Neuropsychology 12: 52–64.

45. Williams J, Phillips T, Griebel M, et al. (2001) Factors associated with academic achievement in children with controlled epilepsy. Epilepsy Behav 2: 217–223.

46. Adams CBT, Beardsworth ED, et al. (1990) Temporal lobectomy in 44 children: Outcome of neuropsychological follow-up. J Epilepsy 3 (Suppl): 157–168.

47. Lendt M, Helmstaedter C, Elger CE. (1999) Pre- and postoperative neuropsychological profiles in children and adolescents with temporal lobe epilepsy. Epilepsia. 40: 1543–1550.

48. Mabbott DM, Smith ML. (2003) Material-specific memory in children with temporal and extratemporal lobectomies. Neuropsychologia. 41: 995–1007.

49. Smith ML, Elliott IM, Lach L. (2004) Cognitive, psychosocial, and family function one year after pediatric epilepsy surgery. Epilepsia 45: 650–660.

50. Szabó CA, Wyllie E, Stanford LD, et al. (1998) Neuropsychological effect of temporal lobe resection in preadolescent children with epilepsy. Epilepsia 39: 814–819.

51. Williams J, Bates S, Griebel ML, et al. (1998) Does short-term antiepileptic drug treatment in children result in cognitive or behavioral changes? Epilepsia. 39: 1064–1069.

52. Helmstaedter C, Kemper B, Elger CE. (1996) Neuropsychological aspects of frontal lobe epilepsy. Neuropsychologia 34: 399–406.

53. Helmstaedter C, Gleissner U, Zentner J, et al. (1998) Neuropsychological consequences of epilepsy surgery in frontal lobe epilepsy. Neuropsychologia 36: 681–689.

54. Upton D, Thompson PJ. (1996) Epilepsy in the frontal lobes: Neuropsychological characteristics. J Epilepsy 9: 215–222.

55. Boone KB, Miller BL, Rosenberg L, et al. (1988) M. Neuropsychological and behavioral abnormalities in an adolescent with frontal lobe seizures. Neurology 38: 583–586.

56. Jambaque I, Dulac O. (1989) Reversible frontal syndrome and epilepsy in an 8-year-old boy. Arch Fr Pediatr 46: 525–529.

57. Blanchette N, Smith ML. (2002) Language after temporal or frontal lobe surgery in children with epilepsy. Brain Cogn 48: 280–284.
58. Culhane-Shelburne K, Chapieski L, Hiscock M, et al. (2002) Executive functions in children with frontal and temporal lobe epilepsy. J Int Neuropsychol Soc 8: 623–632.
59. Hernandez MT, Sauerwein HC, Jambaque I, et al. (2002) Deficits in executive functions and motor coordination in children with frontal lobe epilepsy. Neuropsychologia. 40: 384–400.
60. Lendt M, Gleissner U, Helmstaedter C, et al. (2002) Neuropsychological outcome in children after frontal lobe epilepsy surgery. Epilepsy Behav. 3: 51–59.
61. Nolan MA, Redoblado MA, Lah S, et al. (2004) Memory function in childhood epilepsy syndromes. J Paediatr Child Health 40: 20–27.
62. Riva D, Saletti V, Nichelli F, et al. (2002) Neuropsychologic effects of frontal lobe epilepsy in children. J Child Neurol 17: 661–667.
63. Prevost J, Lortie A, Nguyen D, et al. (2006) Nonlesional frontal lobe epilepsy (FLE) of childhood: Clinical presentation, response to treatment and comorbidity. Epilepsia 47: 2198–2201.
64. Black KC, Hynd GW. (1995) Epilepsy in the school-aged child: cognitive-behavioral characteristics and effects on academic performance. School Psychol Q 10: 345–358.
65. Mitchell W, Lee H, Chavez JM, et al. (1991) Academic underachievement in children with epilepsy. J Child Neurol. 6: 65–72.
66. Seidenberg M. (198) Academic achievement and school performance of children with epilepsy. In: Hermann B, Seidenberg M (eds.) Childhood pilepsies: Neuropsychological, psychosocial and intervention aspects. John Wiley & Sons, Hoboken, NJ: 105–118.
67. Yule, W. (1980) Educational achievement. In: Kulig BM, Meinardi H, Stores G (eds.). Epilepsy and behavior. Lisse, Swets & Zetlinger, The Netherlands: 162–168.
68. Williams J, Sharp GB. (1999) Epilepsy. In: Yeates KO, Ris MD, Taylor HG (eds). Pediatric europsychology. Guilford Press, New York: 47–73.
69. Elliott IM, Lach LM, Smith ML. (2005) "I just want to be normal." A qualitative study exploring how children and adolescents perceive the impact of intractable epilepsy on their quality of life. Epilepsy Behav. 7: 664–678.
70. Thompson PJ. (1987) Educational attainment in children and young people with epilepsy. In:OxleyJ,StoresG (eds.). Epilepsy and education. The Medical Tribune Group, London, 15–24.
71. Austin JK, Huberty TJ, Huster GA, et al. (1998) Academic achievement in children with epilepsy or asthma. Dev Med Child Neurol. 40: 248–255.
72. McNelis AM, Johnson CS, Huberty TJ, et al. (2005) Factors associated with academic achievement in children with recent-onset seizures. Seizure 14: 331–339.
73. Sillanpaa M, Jalava M, Kaleva O, Shinnar S. (1998) Long-term prognosis of seizures with onset in childhood. N Engl J Med 338: 1715–1722.
74. Aldenkamp AP, Alpherts WC, Dekker MJ, et al. (1990) Neuropsychological aspects of learning disabilities in epilepsy. Epilepsia 31 (Suppl 4):9–20.
75. Vermeulen J, Kortsee SWAT, Alpherts WCJ, et al. (1994) Cognitive performance in learning disabled children with and without epilepsy. Seizure 3: 13–21.
76. Sillanpaa M. (2004) Learning disability: Occurrence and long-term consequences in childhood-onset epilepsy. Epilepsy Behav 5: 937–944.
77. Huberty TJ, Austin JK, Risinger MW, et al. (1992) Relationship of selected seizure variables in children with epilepsy to performance on school-administered achievement tests. J Epilepsy. 5: 10–16.
78. Bulteau C, Jambaque I, Viguier D, et al. (2000) Epileptic syndromes, cognitive assessment and school placement: A study of 251 children. Dev Med Child Neurol. 42: 319–327.
79. Vanasse CM, Beland R, Carmant L, et al. (2005) Impact of childhood epilepsy on reading and phonological abilities. Epilepsy Behav. 7: 288–296.
80. Kimura D. (1961) Some effects of temporal-lobe damage on auditory perception. Can J Psychol 15: 156–165.
81. Hermann BP, Seidenberg M, Haltiner A, et al. (1992) Adequacy of language function and verbal memory performance in unilateral temporal lobe epilepsy. Cortex. 8: 423–343.

82. Brockway JP, Follmer RL, Preuss LA, et al. (1998) Memory, simple and complex language, and the temporal lobe. Brain Lang. 61: 1–29.
83. Wagner DD, Sziklas V., Boyle J, et al. (2003) Verbal and visuospatial spans in patients with temporal lobe epilepsy: Critical variables. Epilepsia 44 (Suppl 9): 127
84. Bell B, Dow C, Watson ER, et al. (2003) Narrative and procedural discourse in temporal lobe epilepsy. J Int Neuropsychol Soc 9: 733–739.
85. Milner B. (1990) Right temporal lobe contribution to visual perception and visual memory. In: Iwai E (ed.). Vision, temporal lobe and memory. Elsevier, New York: 43–53.
86. Shields WD. (2004) Diagnosis of infantile spasms, Lennox-Gastaut syndrome, and progressive myoclonic epilepsy. Epilepsia 45 (Suppl 5): 2–4.
87. Dulac O. (1998) Infantile spasms and West syndrome. In: Engel J, Jr, Pedley T (eds.). Epilepsy: A comprehensive textbook, Vol. 3, Lippincott-Raven, Philadelphia 2277–83.
88. Riikonen R. (1996) Long-term outcome of West syndrome: A study of adults with a history of infantile spasms. Epilepsia. 37: 367–372.
89. Riikonen R, Amnell G. (1981) Psychiatric disorders in children with earlier infantile spasms. Dev Med Child Neurol. 23: 747–760.
90. Genton P, Dravet C. (1998) Lennox-Gastaut syndrome and other childhood epileptic encephalopathies. In: Engel J, Jr, Pedley, T (eds.). Epilepsy: A comprehensive textbook, Vol. 3: Lippincott-Raven, Philadelphia 2355–66.
91. Kieffer-Renaux V, Kaminska A, Dulac, O. (2001) Cognitive deterioration in Lennox-Gastaut syndrome and Doos epilepsy. In Jambaque I, Lassonde M, Dulac O (eds.). Neuropsychology of childhood epilepsy. Kluwer Academic/Plenum Publishers, New York: 185–190.
92. Landau WM, Kleffner FR. (1957) Syndrome of acquired aphasia with convulsive disorders in children. Neurology. 7: 523–530.
93. Bishop DV. (1985) Age of onset and outcome in 'acquired aphasia with convulsive disorder' (Landau-Kleffner syndrome) Dev Med Child Neurol. 27: 705–712.
94. Deonna T, Peter C, Ziegler AL. (1989) Adult follow-up of the acquired aphasia-epilepsy syndrome in childhood. Report of 7 cases. Neuropediatrics. 20: 132–138.
95. Casse-Perrot C, Wolf M, Dravet C. (2001) Neuropsychology of severe myoclonic epilepsy in infancy. In: Jambaque I, Lassonde M, Dulac O (eds.). Neuropsychology of childhood epilepsy. Kluwer Academic/Plenum Publishers, New York: 131–140.
96. Dravet C, Bureau M, Guerrini R, et al. (1992) Severe myoclonic epilepsy. In Roger J, Bureau, M, Dravet C, Dreifuss, FE, Perret, A, Wolf M (eds.). Epileptic syndromes in infancy, childhood and adolescence. John Libby Eurotext Ltd., London: 75–88.
97. Motamedi GK, Meador KJ. (2004) Antiepileptic drugs and memory. Epilepsy Behav. 5: 436–439.
98. Ortinski P, Meador KJ. (2004) Cognitive side effects of antiepileptic drugs. Epilepsy Behav 5: S60–S65.
99. Gilliam FG, Fessler AJ, Baker G, et al. (2004) Systematic screening allows reduction of adverse antiepileptic drug effects: A randomized trial. Neurology. 62: 23–27.
100. Meador KJ, Gilliam FG, Kanner AM, Pellock JM. (2001) Cognitive and behavioral effects of antiepileptic drugs. Epilepsy Behav. 2: SS1–SS17.
101. Loring DW, Meador KJ. (2004) Cognitive side effects of antiepileptic drugs in children. Neurology. 62: 872–877.
102. Devinsky O. (1995) Cognitive and behavioral effects of antiepileptic drugs. Epilepsia. 36 (Suppl 2): S46–S65.
103. Trimble MR. (1990) Antiepileptic drugs, cognitive function, and behavior in children: Evidence from recent studies. Epilepsia. 31 (Suppl 4): S30–S34.
104. Vermeulen J, Aldenkamp AP. (1995) Cognitive side effects of chronic antiepileptic drug treatment: A review of 25 years of research. Epilepsy Res 22: 65–95.
105. Meador KJ. (2006) Cognitive and memory effects of the new antiepileptic drugs. Epilepsy Res. 68: 63–67.
106. Martin R, Kuzniecky R, Ho S, et al. (1999) Cognitive effects of topiramate, gabapentin, and lamotrigine in healthy young adults. Neurology. 52: 321–327.

107. Thompson PJ, Baxendale SA, Duncan JS, et al. (2000) Effects of topiramate on cognitive function. J Neurol Neurosurg Psychiat. 69: 636–641.
108. Lee S, Sziklas V, Andermann F, et al. (2003) The effects of adjunctive topiramate on cognitive function inpatients with epilepsy. Epilepsia. 44: 339–347.
109. Aldenkamp AP, Baker G, Mulder OG, et al. (2000) A multicenter randomized clinical study to evaluate the effect on cognitive function of topiramate compared with valproate as add-on therapy to cabamazepine in patients with partial-onset seizures. Epilepsia 41: 1167–1178.
110. Leppick I. (2006) Antiepileptic drug trials in the elderly. Epilepsy Res 68: 45–48.
111. Trimble MR, Cull CA. (1989) Antiepileptic drugs, cognitive function, and behavior in children. Cleve Clin J Med 56 (Suppl 1): S140–S146.
112. Lee DO, Steingard RJ, Cesena M, et al. (1996) Behavioral side effects of gabapentin in children. Epilepsia 37: 87–90.
113. Aarts JHP, Binnie CD, Smith AM. et al. (1984) Selective cognitive impairment during focal and generalized epileptiform EEG activity. Brain 107: 293–308.
114. Siebelink BM, Bakker DJ, Binnie CD, et al. (1988) Psychological effects of subclinical epileptiform EEG discharges in children. II. General intelligence tests. Epilepsy Res 2: 117–121.
115. Hermann B, Seidenberg M, Bell B, et al. (2002) The neurodevelopmental impact of childhood-onset temporal lobe epilepsy on brain structure and function. Epilepsia. 43: 1062–1071.
116. Thompson PJ, Duncan JS. (2005) Cognitive decline in severe intractable epilepsy. Epilepsia 46: 1780–1787.
117. Dodrill CB. (2004) Neuropsychological effects of seizures. Epilepsy Behav 5 (Suppl 1): S21–24.
118. Helmstaedter C, Kurthen M, Lux S, et al. (2003) Chronic epilepsy and cognition: a longitudinal study in temporal lobe epilepsy. Ann Neurol 54: 425–432.
119. Rodin E. (1968) The prognosis of patients with epilepsy. Charles C Thomas. Springfield, IL:
120. Seidenberg M, O'Leary DS, Berent S, et al. (1981) Changes in seizure frequency and test-retest scores on the Wechsler Adult Intelligence Scale. Epilepsia 22: 75–83.
121. Hermann BP, Seidenberg M,Dow C, et al. (2006) Cognitive prognosis in chronic temporal lobe epilepsy. Ann Neurol 60: 80–87.
122. Holmes MD, Dodrill CB, Wilkus RJ, et al. (1998) Is partial epilepsy progressive? Ten-year follow-up of EEG and neuropsychological changes in adults with partial seizures. Epilepsia 39: 1189–1193.
123. Selwa LM, Berent S, Giordani B, et al. (1994) Serial cognitive testing in temporal lobe epilepsy: longitudinal changes with medical and surgical therapies. Epilepsia 35: 743–749.
124. Dodrill CB. (2002) Progressive cognitive decline in adolescents and adults with epilepsy. Prog Brain Res. 135: 399–407.
125. Martin RC, Griffith HR, Faught E, et al. (2005) Cognitive functioning in community dwelling older adults with chronic partial epilepsy. Epilepsia 46: 298–303.
126. Griffith HR, Martin RC, Bambara JK, et al. (2006) Older adults with epilepsy demonstrate cognitive impairments compared with patients with amnestic mild cognitive impairment. Epilepsy Behav 8: 161–168.
127. Piazzini A, Canevini MP, Turner K, et al. (2006) Elderly people and epilepsy: Cognitive function. Epilepsia 47 (Suppl 5): 82–84.

Chapter 13
Nursing and Community Aspects of Epilepsy in Intellectual Disabilities

C. Hanson

Introduction

Epilepsy is defined as "a condition characterized by recurrent epileptic seizures unprovoked by any immediately identified cause."[1] There is an imbalance between excitatory and inhibitory neurons, resulting in excessive excitation or excessive inhibition in specific areas of the cerebral cortex or over the entire cerebral cortex.[2] A person with an intellectual disability (ID) has significant intellectual impairments and deficits in social functioning or adaptive behaviors; onset occurs during the developmental period.[3] The Department of Health[4] acknowledges that people with ID have a significantly reduced ability to understand new or complex information and a reduced ability to cope independently, which starts before adulthood and has a lasting effect on development.

There is no single official statistic that indicates how many people with ID live in the United Kingdom (UK). Government statistics are based on those receiving services and may not include those people who live with their parents or receive no services.

Figures from the National Assembly for Wales[5] identify the following prevalence rates: In the UK the overall prevalence rate for people with severe ID is estimated between 3 and 4 per 1,000 total population, that is, approximately 360–380 per 100,000. It is estimated that there are approximately 10,830 people with severe ID in Wales. The prevalence of mild ID suggests higher rates; approximately 25–30 people per 1,000 total population. In the future, it is estimated that the number of people with severe ID will increase by approximately 1% per year for the next 15 years.[6]

Epilepsy is the most prevalent serious neurological condition in the UK, affecting 1 in 200 people,[7] or 0.5–1% of the general population,[8] and has been highlighted as a national priority for action since 2001.[9] A study carried out in South Wales within a population of 434,000 found that 3,000 patients with epilepsy were identified as alive, giving a period prevalence of 6.9 per 1,000.[10] The prevalence of ID in the general population is approximately similar. Both groups of conditions share a common heritage of heterogeneity, high prevalence figures, and an unfortunate degree of stigmatization.[11]

V.P. Prasher, M.P. Kerr (eds.) *Epilepsy and Intellectual Disabilities*,
DOI: 10.1007/978-1-84800-259-3_13, © Springer Science+Business Media, LLC 2008

There is an increased prevalence of epilepsy in people with ID. Prevalence rates reported in the literature range between 14% and 40%, and the prevalence increases with the greater severity of ID, of up to 50–60%.[12–16] However, the coexistence of epilepsy and ID has been the subject of studies that have used a variety of epidemiological methods and definitions. Inherent population biases have plagued estimates of prevalence of epilepsy in clients with ID. This raises concerns about the estimate of the occurrence of epilepsy in the ID population.[17–18]

Epilepsy is a serious neurological condition that affects people of all ages, races, and social classes. It is often the case that people with ID remain refractory to effective antiepileptic drug treatment.[19] A diagnosis of epilepsy can have far wider implications for the individual. Epilepsy is a condition that carries a social stigma, mainly due to misunderstandings about the condition. People with epilepsy are often discriminated against in such areas as education, employment, and health care.[20] This was highlighted by the National Sentinal Clinical Audit of Epilepsy Related Deaths,[21] which found deficiencies in access to and the quality of care of for people with epilepsy. As a consequence, epilepsy has moved up the health agenda and has been highlighted by a number of organizations, including the British Medical Association, the National Institute for the Clinical Effectiveness, and the National Service Framework (NSF) for Long Term Conditions.[22–24] The proposals within the NSF for improving the care and treatment for people with epilepsy address many of the problems faced in accessing appropriate and timely health and social needs.

These documents have implications for ID services, which are in an ideal position to facilitate the management of epilepsy and people with ID within tertiary care. The epilepsy nurses working within theses teams are easily accessible to clients and already have the core skills and experience of working alongside the psychiatrist and neurologist within epilepsy services and making an important contribution to the management of the person with epilepsy.

Health Care Provision for People with Intellectual Disabilities

The principles of normalization and social role valorization[25–27] state that people with ID should be valued by society. Central to this is the premise of choice and autonomy, or allowing the individual to govern their own lives. This philosophy of care represented the most important single attempt to delabel people with ID. The use of congruence and unconditional positive regard are all key aspects that should be an intrinsic part of health care and a key element to achieving success.

A wealth of published literature discusses obstacles to good health for people with ID and the need to support generic services in order to employ good philosophy of shared practice.[28–30] These documents advocate for social inclusion of people with ID; however, this does not just mean the use of generic services, it also implies providing the proper support to them to access the services they need. As a result, nurses within community ID teams are responding to this inclusive health agenda on a wide range of health needs for people with ID.[31]

Healthcare professionals working in the field of ID have long been aware of this vulnerable group's unmet health needs and the gaps in health care provision for them. Maintaining good levels of general health and well-being is a concern for most people, whether or not they have ID. Since the 1980s, there has been a steady flow of published research articles related to general health and well-being of people with ID. These papers highlight the difficulties people with ID have in accessing health care.[32–36] The publication of "Valuing People: A New Strategy for ID for the 21st Century" clearly highlights the right of people with ID to access a "health service designed around their needs"[37] and also acknowledges wide variations in the quality of health services for people with ID. They recognize the problems of access to health services that some people with ID face, but both clearly expect health promotion initiatives to be part of the work of ID nurses and primary care services as the main providers of health care. They highlighted the need for close collaboration between generic and specialist services.[38] Responses to these government initiatives, local policies, and the change in role from hospital-based care to community care has influenced ID nurses to adapt their practices and evolve new ways of working more than most nurses in other disciplines. The flexible nature of the registered ID nurse is emphasized within the literature. This evidence suggests that the ID nurse is a key person in detecting unmet health needs for people with ID. It has also demonstrated that the community ID nurse is able to make a significant contribution to breaking down some of the many barriers that people with ID face when accessing primary health services.[39–42] The report of the ID nursing project recommended that all primary healthcare workers know when and how to refer clients to ID teams and when to seek advice.[43] The existing evidence, albeit limited, shows that general practitioners are unaware and do not understand the role of ID services.[44] Intellectual disability nurses should be the health facilitators to work in mainstream services to assist in all parts of the National Health Service to develop the necessary skills to enable access to the most appropriate health care to meet the health needs of people with ID.

Unfortunately, even today some public and professional negative attitudes towards people with ID exist, so achieving an ordinary life within the context of ID services is an extraordinary achievement.

Evidence for Change

Since the early 1950s, numerous reports have highlighted the fact that services for people with epilepsy are generally fragmented and poorly coordinated.[45,46] Evidence suggests that people with ID have a lower than average satisfaction with services for epilepsy. There is also little evidence that epilepsy in persons with ID is monitored or reviewed in a primary care setting.

One of the main difficulties is the overall assessment of epilepsy and issues relating to diagnosis among people with ID.[47,48] This is compounded when medical professionals lack the skills needed for communicating with this population.[49–52] Rising concerns regarding the standard of care received generally by people with epilepsy prompted the government to seek advice regarding current service delivery and availability within the UK. The Clinical Standards Advisory Group (CSAG) report outlining epilepsy services in England and Wales suggests that there was no standardized process for care delivery and that the current system for assessment by a general practitioner and referral to a specialist was ad hoc.[53] The report findings also indicated that there is a general lack of access to mainstream epilepsy facilities. However, the survey highlighted the value of having an epilepsy nurse specializing in ID working alongside the psychiatrist. The CSAG made a number of recommendations for improving and increasing equity of services through greater collaboration between specialist centers and for providing better systems for auditing and outcome data collection to support service developments.

Epilepsy Management in Primary Care

Several key studies have highlighted deficiencies in the management of epilepsy within primary care. In 1997, The International League Against Epilepsy, The International Bureau for Epilepsy, and the World Health Organization launched a global campaign to bring epilepsy "out of the shadows" to encourage governments and departments of health to address the needs of people with epilepsy.[54] The National Sentinel Clinical Audit of Epilepsy-Related Death (NSCAERD) examined service provision and aspects of epilepsy management in primary, secondary, and tertiary care. The aim of the audit was to determine whether deficiencies in the standard of care could have contributed towards sudden unexpected death in epilepsy (SUDEP). This finding suggested that approximately 75% of people with epilepsy can achieve effective management of their seizures.[55] The NSCAERD suggests that many of these deaths are associated with seizures and that through appropriate management of the condition the deaths may have been avoided. Within primary care, the main problems highlighted by the audit were lack of appropriate referral and access to specialists, unstructured management plans, and communication failures. As a result of NSCAERD a number of important publications have made recommendations for improving the management of people with epilepsy in primary care. In direct response, "Improving Services for People with Epilepsy"[56] was published. NICE was commissioned to develop guidelines on the diagnosis and management of epilepsy in children and adults and to carry out an appraisal of antiepileptic drugs. The action plan also promotes the inclusion of epilepsy in both the National Service Frameworks for children and for long-term conditions. Furthermore, the action plan recommended that epilepsy be included in contracts for primary care services.[57] In addition to this, a "National Statement of Good Practice, " which outlines the role of general practice in the care of people with epilepsy, was devised.[58]

Evidence suggests that the association between epilepsy and ID has been a neglected field with respect to research, investigation, and guidelines for effective clinical practice. There is little evidence as to the appropriate care provision for people with epilepsy and ID. The delivery of an appropriate standard of care to those people with epilepsy and ID should be guided primarily by an aim to achieve health gain, increase life span, and improve quality of life.[59,60] People with ID and epilepsy have different needs than does the general population. These can be specific to the cause of the ID or to the frequent presence of coexistent behavioral, sensory, or other physical problems. The response to antiepileptic drugs may be less than optimal and less effective than in the non-ID population. Within the clinical setting, difficulties with communication may also require working through a third person, either family or a paid caregiver, and this is a further potential source of difficulty.[61,62] Studies have found rates of behavior disturbance and psychiatric disorder to be significantly higher in people with ID and epilepsy.[63] It is not clear whether this is due to their epilepsy or whether the presence of epilepsy is merely a marker for increased behavioral or psychiatric morbidity.[64] However, it has been suggested that the care of people with ID should be undertaken by a specialist who can work with the multidisciplinary team to ensure seizures can be distinguished from stereotypical and other behavior patterns.[65]

A report from the multidisciplinary primary care project for people with ID and epilepsy highlighted the sense of isolation felt by many caregivers.[66] Many problems arose because lack of information and support from health care professionals, as well as lack of awareness of the help available from various epilepsy associations. There are particular concerns about access to specialist epilepsy services for people with ID. Only 5% of the adults with ID seen in outpatient clinics had evidence that they had seen a specialist with an interest in epilepsy and ID. Further, 6% of adults with ID had been lost to follow-up after transferring to adult care from pediatric services.

Evidence suggests that people with ID and their caregivers do not receive quality service for their epilepsy, and this is confounded by the lack of understanding by healthcare professionals of epilepsy and ID. Increasing that understanding by providing accurate data on frequency and type of seizures, appraising epilepsy-related concerns, and appraising the intrusiveness of the seizures relies heavily upon caregiver support.[67] Crucially, the caregiver's perspective may depend on his or her relationship with the client.[68] Perspectives that caregivers may hold require exploration, because many people with ID have multiple caregivers, who form different types of attachment. Perhaps we should not expect unanimity of opinion or concern, but rather be equipped accurately to appraise a range of expressed needs. Improved communication between primary, secondary, and tertiary services and access to an integrated pathway, shared care protocols, guidelines, and the provision of education and training for staff are paramount to improving services for epilepsy.[69] These include appropriate referral and access to an epilepsy specialist, development of structured management plans, and facilitation of improved communication.

People with ID need the care of the community ID team. The National Institute for Clinical Excellence informing us that "the management and treatment of epilepsy should be undertaken by specialist working within a multi disciplinary team[70]. Epilepsy care for people with ID should achieve a standard that allows these people to live to their full potential. An improvement in the quality of care is required and the individual's perspective should remain central.

The Epilepsy Specialist Nurse

The epilepsy specialist nurse's role should be a fundamental element of a multidisciplinary epilepsy team. He or she works alongside specialists and generalists and plays a part in the assessment and diagnostic process, establishing the quality of life impact on the patient as well as giving advice and support.[71,72] Patients with epilepsy often find it difficult to obtain support when they need it and will require adequate and appropriate information about how to deal with their epilepsy. The specialist nurse is often the best person to acknowledge the patient's fears. The epilepsy specialist nurse may triage undiagnosed or newly referred clients following a first seizure, take a medical history, consider the differential diagnosis, initiate and interpret diagnostic investigations in consultation with consultant colleagues. Clients with refractory epilepsy are monitored for antiepileptic drug efficacy and side effects; some epilepsy specialist nurses who are independent prescribers advise clients on medication changes to improve treatment.[73,74]

Nurse-Led Epilepsy Clinics

Although numerous publications have examined the effectiveness of nurse-led epilepsy clinics, they all tend to focus on secondary care.[75–80] The majority of the literature exploring nurse-led clinics tends to be found within the popular nursing press and often extends to only a few pages. There are very few studies that have examined the effectiveness of nurse-led epilepsy clinics within primary care and tertiary care. Such papers tend to be highly positive regarding the clinics, but are generally descriptive and lack the deeper analysis which provides insight into how and why the clinic has developed.

The UK government has acknowledged the concept of specialist nurses.[81] "The government is particularly keen to extend developments in the role of nurses working in community services…taking on leadership roles, monitoring and educating nurses and other staff, managing care, developing nurse led clinics across organisational and professional boundaries ensuring continuity and integration of care." The latest clinical guidelines for the management of epilepsy in children and adults recommend that each epilepsy team should include epilepsy specialist nurses. The National Institute for Clinical Excellence makes a similar recommendation: "epilepsy specialist nurses should be an integral part of the network of care of individuals with epilepsy."[82,83]

Evidence suggests that it is the ID nurse who provides the cohesive link between the person with ID and epilepsy and everyone providing care. The ID epilepsy nurse is an asset to community due to their dual qualifications and training. Within the United Kingdom it is through a link with the community ID nurse that community epilepsy management should ideally occur.[84–85]

The natural progression for epilepsy nursing within community-based nursing is the development of nurse-led epilepsy clinics, following a template similar to asthma and diabetic clinics.[86] A plethora of documents exist to guide professionals in developing epilepsy services, but in order to maximize and extend these theories into the ID field, there needs to be an experienced practitioner driving the development of clinical services.

Nurse-led care reflects a model of service in which nurses have a higher profile in providing care based on their own assessment of the client's needs. Such decisions are based on the nurse's level of skill and ability and their interpretation of the scope of practice.

There is increasing evidence that nurse-led clinics are comparable and, in some cases, better in terms of patient satisfaction, quality, and cost than those that are medically led. Improving epilepsy services within primary and secondary care is to increase the number of epilepsy specialist nurses. Several other studies suggest that the tangible benefits of patient access to a specialist epilepsy nurse included improved cost effectiveness, a reduction in the length of a hospital stay, increased patient satisfaction, and enhanced drug compliance.[87,88] However, patients are generally satisfied with their overall care. Young people and people with severe epilepsy preferred hospital care, while older patients preferred primary care. Some patients reported gains at a cognitive and affective level from the nurse intervention. They linked learning to the nurse's approach of inquiring about lifestyle issues and providing information responsively.[89]

A recent study tested the feasibility and effect of nurse-run clinics in general practice.[90] The study consists of a randomized-controlled trial of nurse-run clinics versus "usual care" in six general practices in the South Thames region. The overall conclusions from the investigation were that nurse-run clinics were feasible and well attended; the study highlighted significant improvements in the level of advice recorded (drug therapy, treatment compliance, and lifestyle issues). Ways in which drug management could be improved were identified in one fifth of the patients. Another study compared patients' assessments of the care provided by their general practitioner, neurologist, and the epilepsy specialist nurse based within secondary care. The outcome of the studies concluded that patients expressed greater satisfaction with the care provided by the epilepsy specialist nurse in areas such as information, advice, counselling, and continuity of care.[91,92] By improving communication and satisfaction, epilepsy specialist nurses can improve the health status of patients with epilepsy and reduce the waiting lists for consultants.

One of the most frightening aspects of epilepsy for clients and their caregivers is a lack of control. Providing clients with ID and their caregivers with user-friendly and inclusive information to enable them to understand their condition helps remove the myths and reduce the fear surrounding the condition and also helps to empower clients to take more control over their epilepsy.[92,93] Most clients with epilepsy would like more information about their condition and would prefer to discuss their condition with a nurse, as nurses were found to be empathic and to have more time for clinic appointments.[94]

Comparable improvements in satisfaction and patient management have also been reported in two qualitative reports on epilepsy nurse intervention.[95,96] Through the establishment of a nurse-led clinic, nurse specialists contributed towards improved counselling, support, and education to clients and their families. An improved understanding of epilepsy and its treatment could lead indirectly to an improved quality of life for clients and their families.

Specific Components of the Specialist Epilepsy Nurse's Role

Epilepsy specialist nurses have an important role in supporting the overall management of epilepsy in persons with ID. The individual management of epilepsy is essential given that epilepsy impacts people in many different ways. The NICE guidelines state that each person should have a comprehensive care plan, including medical and lifestyle issues, that is agreed upon by the individual and the primary, secondary, or tertiary services. The epilepsy specialist nurse will undertake an initial assessment and complete an epilepsy profile, which is an essential component to support a diagnosis and treatment plan. A person-centered approach is fundamental in supporting the person with epilepsy to lead an independent life with as few restrictions as possible.

The following are the key components of the role:

- Provide effective specialist nursing skills, knowledge, and expertise in the care and management of people with intellectual disabilities and epilepsy
- Supplementary and Independent Nurse prescribing
- Facilitate nurse-led clinics: Triage, Transition, Vagus Nerve Stimulation
- Undertake a holistic epilepsy assessment and plan patient-centered care
- Coordinate partnership working between health care and social services and other agencies
- Encourage the individual to keep a seizure diary
- Completion of an epilepsy profile with individual epilepsy management guidelines/rescue medication guidelines
- Determine the correct diagnosis of epilepsy and assist in the detailed investigation of differential diagnosis
- Define seizure types and seizure syndromes
- Discuss symptomatic focal seizures and possibility of surgery. Offer concise information on trial results, VNS, surgery, etc.
- Initiate consideration of specialized drug treatments for complex seizure management and syndromic diagnosis
- Provide support and guidance to clients and cares through complex medication titration regimens
- Monitor concordance of medication

- Assess and initiate risk assessments for the person with epilepsy
- Identify subtle changes through the understanding of the pathology and presentation of the epilepsy and its effect on cognitive function
- Recognize and monitor potential complications from polypharmacy, drug side effects, behavioral changes, and cognitive decline
- Identify health problems and physical difficulties which affect behavior and epilepsy
- Provide education and information to people with epilepsy and their families
- Provide preconception counseling to women of child-bearing age
- Develop and participate in educational protocols, standards, and guidelines
- Participate in clinical reviews
- Provide flexible services to support people to live independently at home
- Liaise with secondary care to improve inpatient care
- Evaluate quality of life and other clinical outcomes
- Audit and research

People with Intellectual Disabilities and Assessing Risks in Epilepsy

People with epilepsy and ID live in various care settings and are supported by either families or provider agencies or live independently in their own homes. The level of risk will depend upon each individual, the frequency, severity of their epilepsy, and the environment surrounding them at the time of the seizure.[97] It is important to assess the level of risk in order to reduce psychosocial morbidity and the impact of the seizures on the individual's quality of life. This management as part of an integrated care pathway can be coordinated by the epilepsy specialist nurse, who will link into a multidisciplinary team that includes psychiatry, psychology, speech and language therapy, occupational therapy, and dietetics and undertake the respective risk assessment. The aimes of the pathway being to:-

- To reduce seizure-related morbidity: head injuries, burns, scalds
- To reduce seizure-related mortality: SUDEP, drowning, and accidents
- To reduce treatment-related morbidity: monitoringside effects of medication, medication concordance, cognitive impairment.
- To reduce psychosocial morbidity: reduce overprotection, encourage participation in social activities, and activities of daily living.

Consent

It is a general legal and ethical principle that valid consent must be obtained before starting any treatment or physical intervention.[98,99] For a person to have capacity, he or she must be able to comprehend and retain information in relation to the pending decision. If the person lacks capacity, a key principle concerning treatment is that of the person's best interests. It is good practice for the multidisciplinary team to involve those close to the person to be able to demonstrate that any treatment offered is in that person's best interests.

When people with ID undergo a general anesthetic for a brain scan, the surgical team will not proceed unless the consent forms are signed. The epilepsy specialist nurse is in a key position to liaise with the person and professionals involved to establish a care pathway that will facilitate the systematic process of care between services.

Women and Epilepsy

Women with ID should be treated the same as any other women and be offered preconception counseling, both to control their seizures and to make sure that their contraception, fertility, pregnancies, fetal development, childcare, and eventual menopause are not compromised either by the epilepsy itself or by the medication needed to control the seizures. Evidence suggests that referral to an epilepsy specialist nurse for preconception counseling can be beneficial. The nurse should be available and supportive throughout the process to answer questions and enable the women and their caregivers to make an informed decision regarding the choices available to her.[100]

Contraception

According to best practice guidelines for the management of women with epilepsy, preconception counseling should start at the time of diagnosis and be repeated at intervals throughout the management.[101] A diagnosis of epilepsy and treatment with antiepileptic drugs present women of child bearing age with particular problems. Phenobarbitone, primidone, carbamazepine, and topiramate are inducers of the hepatic P-450 microsomal isoenzyme which is responsible for the metabolism of estrogens and progestrogens[102] and therefore reduces contraceptive efficacy. Lamotrigine may also reduce the efficacy of the combined oral contraceptive pill (COC), but the evidence is limited and conflicting. The COC is usually prescribed at 50mcg daily. In addition, the COC induces the metabolism by up to 2–3 times, lowering the lamotrigine levels so that a higher dose may be needed.[103] Conversely, when stopping the COC, the dose of lamotrigine may need to be reduced to prevent the drug rising to toxic levels. Another contraceptive alternative would be to consider the depot provera given at 10 weekly intervals instead of 12 weekly intervals.

Pregnancy

During pregnancy, plasma levels of lamotrigine fall. It is good practice to obtain baseline lamotrigine levels and during pregnancy monitor levels which will support clinical decisions. If an increased dose is required during pregnancy, it should be remembered that the dose may need to be lowered after pregnancy, as levels may become toxic. Folic acid supplementation during pregnancy reduces the risk of spina bifida, especially if the woman is taking enzyme-inducing medication.

Menstruation and Catamenial Epilepsy

Evidence suggests that a proportion of women with active epilepsy will experience an increase in seizure activity around their menstrual cycle. When measured accurately, only 12% of women have a definite time relationship between seizure occurrence and their menstrual cycle.[104] Estrogen is mildly epileptogenic, and the high estrogen concentration in the follicular phase of the menstrual cycle is a possible underlying cause for the greater propensity of seizures. Seizures may respond, however, to intermittent "rescue" medication such as clobazam.[105,106]

Genetics

The genetics white paper outlines how advances in knowledge and understanding are bringing more accurate diagnosis, more personalized prediction of risk, new drugs and therapies, better targeted preventions and treatment of disease informed by an individual's genetic profile.[107] Developments in epilepsy genetic syndromes continue to provide opportunities for more accurate diagnosis of rare epilepsy syndromes. They may also provide more insight in to the genetic component and environmental triggers of common conditions. Being able to provide a more accurate diagnosis will also help in deciding which services may be needed to support a patient and his or her family. Parents of children and adults referred for genetic counseling require support from the epilepsy specialist nurse as well as from regional genetic services.[108,109]

Conclusion

Epilepsy is a chronic disorder, and people with an ID and epilepsy must try to understand the complexities of their condition. Being diagnosed with epilepsy involves learning to deal with the physical impact of the seizure, as well as the medical and surgical management of them. Although the assessment of epilepsy in people with an ID do not differ from general services, it is important that an epilepsy pathway is followed that maps a process of care enabling professionals, patients, and caregivers to have a clear focus of the care expected . Most people with an ID rely on others to identify and communicate their symptoms to health professionals. Epilepsy nurse involvement as lead health professional demonstrates the significant contributions nurses within community services are making to the management of epilepsy care. Person-centered and person-directed treatment are both essential to enable people with epilepsy to maintain a good quality of life and manage the psychosocial consequences of seizures which can impact significantly on their daily life.

References

1. Smithson. (2000) Epilepsy in primary care. Primary Health Care 10:18–21.
2. Hickey J. (2003) The clinical practice of neurological and neurosurgical nursing. Philadelphia: Lippincott, Williams and Williams.
3. American Association on Mental Retardation. (2002) Mental retardation – definition classification and system of supports (AAMR), 10th ed. Washington DC.
4. Department of Health. (2001) Shifting the balance of power within the NHS securing delivery. London: HMSO.
5. National Assembly for Wales. (2001) Fulfilling the promises: A proposal for a framework for services for people with learning disabilities. Cardiff: NAW.
6. Department of Health. (2001) Valuing people: A new strategy for learning disability for the 21st century. London: HMSO.
7. National Society for Epilepsy. (2004) London.
8. Morgan C, Kerr M. (2001) The epidemiology of epilepsy revisited. Ann Neurol 49:336–344.
9. Epilepsy Action. (2005) Epilepsy facts, figures and terminology. http://www.epilepsy.org. uk/uk/press/facts.html
10. Morgan C, Kerr M. (2002) Epilepsy and mortality: A record linkage study in a UK population. Epilepsia 43: 1251–1255.
11. Lhatoo S, Sander J. (2001) The epidemiology of epilepsy and learning disability. Epilepsia 42: 6–9.
12. Bowley C, Kerr M. (2000) Epilepsy and intellectual disability. J Intellect Dis Res 44: 529–543.
13. International Association of the Scientific Study of Intellectual Disabilities (IASSID). (2001) Clinical guidelines for the management of epilepsy in adults with an intellectual disability. Seizure 10: 401–409.
14. Crawford P, Brown S, Kerr M. (2001) A randomized open-label study of gabapentin and lamotrigine in adults with learning disability and resistant epilepsy. Seizure 10: 107–115.
15. Sheepers M, Kerr M. (2003) Epilepsy and behaviour. Neurology 16: 183–187.
16. Deb S, Joyce J. (1999) The use of antiepileptic medication in a population-based cohort of adults with learning disability and epilepsy. Int J Psych Clin Practice 3: 1–5.
17. Welsh Office. (1995) Welsh health survey. Cardiff: Welsh Office.
18. Kerr M, Bowley C. (2001) Multidisciplinary and multiagency contributions to care for those with learning disability who have epilepsy. Epilepsia 42: 5–56.
19. Smithson WH. (2000) Epilepsy in primary care. Primary Health Care 10: 18–21.
20. Clarke B, Upton A, Castellanos C. (2006) Work beliefs and work status in epilepsy. Epilepsy Behav 9: 119–125.
21. Hannah J, Black M, Sander J, et al. (2002) The national sentinel clinical audit of epilepsy related death: Epilepsy — Death in the shadows. London: The Stationary Office.

22. British Medical Association. (2004) New general medical services contract. BMA. London:
23. National Institute for Clinical Excellence. (2004) The epilepsies: Diagnosis and management of the epilepsies in adults in primary and secondary care. London: NICE.
24. Department of Health. (2005) National service framework for long term conditions. London: HMSO.
25. Wolfensberger W. (1972) The principles of normalisation in human services. Toronto: National Institute on Mental Retardation.
26. Wolfensberger W. (1983) Social role valorisation: A proposed new term for the principle of normalisation. Mental Retard 21: 234–239.
27. O'Brien J. (1987) A guide to lifestyle planning: using the activities to integrate services and natural support systems. In: Wilcox BW, Bellamy GT. The activities catalogue: An alternative for youth and adults with severe disabilities. Baltimore: PH Brookes.
28. Gates B. (2003) Learning disabilities: Toward inclusion, 4th ed. Churchill Livingstone. London:
29. Department of Health. (1998) Signposts to success in commissioning and providing health services for people with learning disabilities. London: NHS Executive.
30. Department of Health. (1999) Making a difference. Strengthening the nursing, midwifery and health visiting contribution to health and healthcare. London: HMSO.
31. Department of Health. (2001) Shifting the balance of power within the NHS securing delivery. London: HMSO.
32. Corbett J, Thomas C, Prior M, et al. (2003) Health facilitation for people with learning disabilities. Br J Comm Nursing 8: 405–410.
33. Howells G (1996) Situations vacant: Doctors required to provide care for people with learning disabilities. Br J Gen Practice 46: 59–60.
34. Williams R, Rhead L. (2003) Community learning disability nursing. In: Watkins W, Edwards J, Gastrell P (eds.). Community health nursing: Frameworks for practice. London: Bailliere Tindall.
35. Cumella S, Martin D. (2002) Secondary care for people with a learning disability. Br Inst Learning Disability. London: BILD.
36. Gibson T. (2006) Welcoming the learning disabled practice. Practice Nursing 17: 593–596.
37. Kerr M. (2006) Reducing the impact of epilepsy in people with a learning disability. Prog Neurol Psychiat 10: 20–26.
38. Department of Health. (2003) Improving services for people with epilepsy. Action Plan. London: DOH.
39. Powrie E. (2001) Caring for adults with a learning disability. Br J Nursing 10: 928–939.
40. Beacock C. (2001) Come in from the cold. Nursing Standard 15: 23.
41. Gates B. (2003) Learning disabilities: Toward inclusion, 4th ed. Churchill Livingstone. London:
42. Davies D, Northway R. (2001) Collaboration in primary care. J Comm Nursing 15: 14–18.
43. Hunt C, Flecknor D, King M, et al. (2004) Access to secondary care for people with learning disabilities. Nursing Times 100: 34–36.
44. Bollard M. (1999) Learning disability nursing: Improving primary care for people with learning disabilities. Br J Nursing 8: 1216–1221.
45. British Epilepsy Association. (2000) An agenda for action. Leeds: BEA.
46. Brown S. (1999) A two year follow up of NHS executive letter 95/120. Where is the commitment to equality? Seizure 8: 128–131.
47. Bradley P. (1998) Audit of epilepsy services in Northamptonshire Health Authority.
48. Jenkins L, Brown S. (1996) Some issues in the assessment of epilepsy occurring in the context of learning disability in adults. Seizure 1: 49–55.
49. Singh P. (1997) Prescription for change: Mencap report on the role of GP's and carers in the provision of primary care for people with learning disabilities. London: Mencap.
50. Thornton C. (1999) Effective healthcare for people with learning disabilities: A formal carers' perspective. J Psych Ment Health Nursing 6: 383–390.
51. Espie C. (1998) The epilepsy outcome scale: The development of a measure for use with carers of people with epilepsy plus intellectual disability. J Intellect Dis Res 42: 90–96.
52. Kerr M, Todd S. (1996) Caring together in epilepsy. Issues in the care of people with learning disabiliti es and epilepsy. Cardiff: The Welsh Centre for Learning Disabilities.

53. Department of Health. (2000) Services for patients with epilepsy. The Stationary Office. London: Report of a clinical standards Advisory Group (CSAG) committee chaired by Professor Alison Kitson.

54. Reynolds E. (2002) Epilepsy in the world: Launch of the second phase of the ILAE/IBE/ WHO global campaign against epilepsy. Epilepsia 43: 6.

55. Epilepsy Action. (2005) Epilepsy facts, figures and terminology. http://www.epilepsy.org. uk/uk/press/facts.html

56. Department of Health. (2003) New roles for nurses and GPs to expand primary care and drive down waiting lists. http://www.dh.gov.uk/publicationsandstatistics/pressreleases/pressreleasesnotices/

57. British Medical Association. (2004) New general medical services contract. London: BMA.

58. Joint Epilepsy Council. (2002) National statement of good practice for the treatment and care of people who have epilepsy. Liverpool: JEC.

59. Bowley C, Kerr M. (2000) Epilepsy and intellectual disability. J Intellect Dis Res 44: 529–543.

60. Kerr M, Bowley C. (2001) Multidisciplinary and multiagency contributions to care for those with learning disability who have epilepsy. Epilepsia 42: 55–56.

61. Kacperek L. (1997) Non-verbal communication: The importance of listening. Br J Nursing 6: 275–279.

62. Van der Gaag A. (1998) Communication skills and adults with learning disabilities: Eliminating professional myopia Br J Learning Disabil 26: 88–93.

63. Bouras N, Drummond C. (1992) Behaviour and psychiatric disorders of people with mental handicaps living in the community. J Intellect Dis Res 36: 349–357.

64. Deb S. (1997) Mental disorder in adults with mental retardation and epilepsy. Compr Psychiat 38: 179–184.

65. Shuttleworth A. (2004) Implementing new guidelines on epilepsy management. Nursing Times 100: 28–29.

66. Frith A. (1997) Improving health of people with learning disabilities living in the community. The Halton Learning Disabilities Project. North Cheshire Health.

67. Kerr M, Espie C. (2002) Epilepsy and learning disability. Implications for quality of life. In: Epilepsy. Beyond seizure counts in assessment and treatment. In: Baker G, Jacoby A (eds.). Amsterdam: Harwood Academic Publishers.

68. Espie C, Watkins J, Duncan R, et al. (2003) Perspectives on epilepsy in people with intellectual disabilities: Comparison of family carer, staff carer and clinical score profiles on the Glasgow Epilepsy Outcome Scale (GEOS). Seizure 12: 195–202.

69. Hayes C. (2004) Clinical skills: Practical guide for managing adults with epilepsy. Br J Nursing 13: 7–10.

70. National Institute for Clinical Excellence. (2004) The epilepsies: Diagnosis and management of the epilepsies in adults in primary and secondary care. NICE, London: 37.

71. Scottish Intercollegiate Guidelines Network. (2003) Diagnosis and management of epilepsy in adults. Edinburgh: SIGN.

72. Risdale L, Kwan I, Morgan M. (2003) How can a nurse intervention help people with newly diagnosed epilepsy? A qualitative study of patients' views. Seizure 12: 69–73.

73. Mills N, Bachmann M, Cambell R, et al. (1999) Effect of a primary care based epilepsy service on quality of care from a patients perspective: Results at two years follow-up. Seizure 8: 291–296.

74. Macdonald D, Torrance N, Wood S, et al. (2000) General-practice-based nurse specialists-- taking a lead in improving the care of people with epilepsy. Seizure 9: 31–35.

75. Hatchett R. (2003) Nurse led clinics: Practice issues. Routledge. London:

76. Poole K, Moran N, Bell G. (2000) Patients' perspectives on services for epilepsy: A survey of patient satisfaction, preference and information provision in 2394 people with epilepsy. Seizure 9: 551–558.

77. Risdale L. (2000) The effect of a specially trained epilepsy nurses in primary care: A review. Seizure9:43–46.

78. Mills N, Campbell R, Bachmann M. (2002) Professional and organizational obstacles to establishing a new specialist service in primary care. Case study of an epilepsy specialist nurse. J Adv Nursing 37(1): 43–51.

79. Rogers D, Taylor M. (1996) Don't fit in front of your work mates: Living with epilepsy in Doncaster. Doncaster: Doncaster Medical Audit Advisory Group.
80. Rogers G. (2003) Emerging guidance for epilepsy: The onus on primary care professionals to have an increased awareness of epilepsy issues. Primary Health Care 13 (6): 39–42.
81. Department of Health. (1997) The new NHS. London: HMSO.
82. National Institute for Clinical Excellence. (2004) The epilepsies: Diagnosis and management of the epilepsies in adults in primary and secondary care. NICE, London: 37.
83. Scottish Intercollegiate Guidelines Network. (2003) Diagnosis and management of epilepsy in adults. Edinburgh: SIGN.
84. Hannah J, Brodie M. (1998) Epilepsy and learning disabilities — a challenge for the next millennium? Seizure 7: 3–13.
85. Kerr M. (2003) Fraser W, Kerr M. Epilepsy in the psychiatry of learning disabilities. In: 2nd ed. London: The Royal College of Psychiatrists.
86. Rogers G. (2003) Emerging guidance for epilepsy: The onus on primary care professionals to have an increased awareness of epilepsy issues. Primary Health Care 13 (61): 39–42.
87. Hatchett R. (2003) Nurse led clinics: Practice Issues. London: Routledge.
88. Poole K, Moran N, Bell G, et al. (2000) Patients' perspectives on services for epilepsy: A survey of patient satisfaction, preference and information provision in 2394 people with epilepsy. Seizure 9: 551–558.
89. Risdale L, Robins D, Cryer C, et al. (1997) Feasibility and effects of nurse run clinics for patients with epilepsy in general practice: Randomised controlled trial. Br Med J314: 120–122.
90. Scrambler A, Scrambler G, Risdale L, et al. (1996) Towards an evaluation of the effectiveness of an epilepsy nurse in primary care. Seizure 5: 255–258.
91. Goodwin M, Higgins S, Lanfear J, et al. (2004) The role of the clinical nurse specialist in epilepsy in the United Kingdom. Epilepsia 43: 8.
92. Epilepsy Advisory Board. (1999) Epilepsy care: Making it happen. A toolkit for today. London: Epilepsy Advisory Board.
93. Scrambler A, Scrambler G, Risdale L, Robins D. (1996) Towards an evaluation of the effectiveness of an epilepsy nurse specialist in primary care. Seizure 5: 255–258.
94. Higgins S. (2006) Quantifying the role of nurse specialists in epilepsy. Data from diaries and interviews. Br J Neurosci Nursing 2 (5): 239–246.
95. Taylor M, Readman S, Hague B, Boulter V, Hughes L, Howells S. (1994) A district epilepsy service, with community based specialist liaison nurse and guidelines for shared care. Seizure 3: 121–127.
96. Appleton R, Sweeney E. (1995) The management of epilepsy in children: The role of the clinical nurse specialist. Seizure 4: 287–291.
97. International Association of the Scientific Study of Intellectual Disabilities (IASSID). (2001) Clinical guidelines for the management of epilepsy in adults with an intellectual disability. Seizure 10: 401–409.
98. National Assembly for Wales. (2002) Reference guide to consent for examination or treatment. Cardiff: NAW.
99. British Medical Association and the Law Society. (1995) Assessment of mental capacity: Guidance for doctors and lawyers. London: BMA Publishing Group.
100. Greenhill L, Betts T. (2003) The lifelong care needs of women with epilepsy. Practice Nursing 14 (7): 302–309.
101. Crawford P. (2005) Best practice guidelines for the management of women with epilepsy. Epilepsia 46 (9): 117–124.
102. Craig J. (2005) Epilepsy and women. In: Saunder J, Walker M, Smalls J (eds.). Epilepsy 2005, from euron to NICE: A practical guide, 10th ed. St. Annes College. Oxford: Lecture notes for the 10th epilepsy teaching weekend.
103. Sabers A, Bucholt J, Uldall P, Hansen E. (2001) Lamotrigine plasma levels reduced by oral contraceptives Epilepsy Res 47: 151–154.
104. Svalheim S, Tauboll E, Bjornenak T, Morland T. (2006) Onset of epilepsy and menarche — Is there any relationship? Seizure 15: 571–575.

105. Shorvon S. (2000) Handbook of epilepsy treatment. London: Blackwell Science.
106. Betts T, Crawford P. (1998) Women and epilepsy. London: Martin Dunitz.
107. Department of Health. (2003) Our inheritance, our future. Realising the potential of genetics in the NHS. London: The Stationary Office.
108. Barr O, Miller R. (2003) Parents of children with intellectual disabilities, their expectations and experience of genetic counseling. J Applied Res Intellectual Disabil. 16: 189–204.
109. Skirton H. (2001) The client's perspective of genetic counseling — a grounded theory study. J Genet Counseling 10 (4): 311–329.

Chapter 14
Epilogue – Is This as Good as it Gets?

M.P. Kerr and V.P. Prasher

If professionals and caregivers assimilated and practiced the body of knowledge presented in this work, it is likely that many people with epilepsy would experience an improvement in the quality of their lives. However, this would still leave many with a very considerable seizure disorder and associated restricted social inclusion. The question we would like to finish with is, Is this level of improvement as good as it gets for people with intellectual disability and epilepsy? We therefore propose three interconnected aspirations for the future of epilepsy care for people with an intellectual disability: *universal access to specialized epilepsy services, seizure freedom, and an absence of epilepsy-related social restriction.*

Universal access to specialized care should surely be obtainable; however, major barriers need to be removed for this to occur. The first is lack of education and recognition of the real needs of this population, which results in a tendency to underestimate (and underfund) need. It is unusual to meet a person with intellectual disability and epilepsy who could not benefit from change in some aspect of their care, yet all too often this population is left to languish in services unprepared to refer for change or to change the epilepsy management itself. The approach to redress this situation should involve empowerment of individuals and their caregivers and direct auditable standards of care within both primary and secondary care. Where the health system is target driven, these targets should be meaningful and linked to health gain. The second is misplacement of philosophical aspirations – an ordinary life means an ordinary outcome in life, which may need very special help to be achieved. Epilepsy services for this population should reflect these needs. The current setup of very brief review for the majority of people in primary care will simply not meet the needs of this population. Likewise a policy of generic care will restrict some patients' access to skilled learning disability services that are aware of, and capable of approaching, the complex needs of this population. Furthermore, such a generic policy will undermine efforts to deliver care in nonlearning disability services. Lastly, political and professional prioritization is needed. This is particularly important in a population whose voice is so rarely heard.

Seizure freedom for all may seem unrealistic. It remains a crucial aspiration. The scientific basis to achieve this aim is constantly advancing. New methodologies in neuroimaging, such as magnetoencephalograms and increased power of MRI scanners,

V.P. Prasher, M.P. Kerr (eds.) *Epilepsy and Intellectual Disabilities*,
DOI: 10.1007/978-1-84800-259-3_14, © Springer Science+Business Media, LLC 2008

have advanced our ability to identify specific brain lesions and increase access to surgical options. Pharmacological advances continue to make slow but definite progress through identifying new targets for AEDs or through producing drugs with improved tolerability.

While these improvements will chip away at seizure freedom, it may be through advances in our ability to understand individuals that the most major changes will be made. These advances have been mainly in the field of genetics and molecular biology. While individual variation in response to treatment has been an integral part of epilepsy management – as seen by one individual's ability to tolerate large doses of an AED and another's inability to tolerate even the smallest dose – we have had little idea why this is. Recent advances in understanding how drugs are transported into the brain, through a system known as Multi Drug Resistance Proteins, have identified a potential identifiable mechanism to target for accurate drug dosing. Researchers have shown that individual genetic variation in the expression of these proteins influences the transport of AEDs into the brain -- possibly explaining "resistance" to drugs in some individuals. The next major advance in understanding individuals comes through the recognition of the causation of intellectual disability. This explosion in genetic knowledge holds out hope that the specific causation may either match to a particular type of treatment due to its mode of action or in some cases through the ability to treat the individual cause. Although actually reversing the process which can lead to the development of the epilepsy remains a distant dream, recent work showing that aspects of the Rett phenotype expressed in Rett Mice acts as a proof that such reversibility may be possible.

The removal of *epilepsy-related social restriction* poses a completely different set of hurdles. Medical advance will exclude some of these through removal of seizures or through improved treatment of acute seizures. Unfortunately, lessons from studies in people with epilepsy who do not have an intellectual disability suggest that removal of seizures does not lead in itself to complete removal of the stigma associated with epilepsy. Notwithstanding this, epilepsy is slowly moving "out of the shadows," and this move will help people with an intellectual disability. Public education, the identification of role models with epilepsy, backed up by an antidiscriminatory legal framework, will go some way toward reducing social restriction.

No part of medicine exists in isolation of others, and while people with intellectual disability who have epilepsy are rarely prioritized in research, they will gain much from the advances made across science as a whole. The future may not be perfect, but it does hold hope. The task for those committed to this population is to ensure that a voice can be heard that recognizes not just the importance of this group, but also how meeting its special needs and special challenges will enhance the care of all.

Index